Culturally Responsive Substance Use Treatment

This book invites readers into the transformative world of culturally responsive substance use treatment and illuminates the importance of integrating cultural understanding and sensitivity into every aspect of substance use treatment, offering a comprehensive guide for organizations, practitioners, and students alike.

Drawing from her extensive experience in the industry, Dr. Jones masterfully articulates why cultural responsiveness is critical when providing substance use treatment. She skillfully delves into the intricate ways in which culture influences an individual's relationship with substance use, emphasizing the need for tailored and inclusive interventions. Through compelling case studies, practical tools, and thought-provoking insights, Dr. Jones empowers readers to navigate the complexities of culture, paving the way for more effective and impactful treatment strategies utilizing her developed framework.

This book is an indispensable resource for anyone seeking to transform the landscape of substance use treatment and promote equitable, inclusive care.

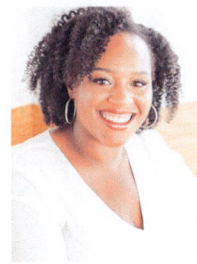

Gabrielle Jones, Ph.D., is a licensed psychologist and the CEO of Steady Clinical Consultation, Training, and Development Services. She completed her Ph.D. in Counseling Psychology at Oklahoma State University. She has over a decade of experience teaching and providing culturally responsive substance use treatment at all treatment levels and life stages. Dr. Jones Also received the American Society of Addiction Medicine's (ASAM) 2024 DEI in Addiction Medicine Award.

"Our relationship with substances is, well, complicated. Depending on the societal perspective of the day, any given substance could be a detriment to society, a burgeoning industry, or somewhere on that spectrum. In *Culturally Responsive Substance Use Treatment: A Guide for Practitioners, Students, and Organizations*, Dr. Gabrielle Jones takes on the historical and contemporary issues while offering timely and relevant insight into the culture, more broadly, and the often overlooked and marginalized subcultures. She offers a fresh voice that makes this book impactful for all types of readers. Dr. Jones's fusion of issues, coupled with her penchant for truth-telling, makes this book a must-read."

Donell Barnett, Ph.D., *past president,*
The Association of Black Psychologists

"This is a fabulous book! Jones offers a treasure trove of practical advice, clinically relevant suggestions, and deep insights based on her extensive clinical experience and knowledge. Case examples are diverse and nuanced, with rich explanations of the historical reasons for practices that have become outdated. I expect this text will become *the* go-to source for culturally responsive substance use treatment!"

Pamela A. Hays, Ph.D., *licensed psychologist*
and creator of the ADDRESSING framework

"Dr. Gabrielle Jones is a beacon of hope for the fields of psychology and addiction medicine, shining a light on the inequities in patient care perpetuated by the systemic oppression of BIPOC communities. She eloquently guides the reader through the problems with our current frameworks of culturally competent substance use treatment and offers concrete solutions for professionals and leaders. Dr. Jones is revolutionizing mental health and addiction services at a time when the world so desperately needs support. "Culturally Responsive Substance Use Treatment: A Guide for Practitioners, Students, and Organizations" should be a required reading for all graduate students, healthcare providers, and industry leaders."

Jessica Byrd Olmstead, Ph.D., *licensed psychologist,*
entrepreneur, addiction and adolescent expert

"Dr. Gabrielle Jones has provided a nuanced understanding of substance use and substance abuse treatment. Dr. Jones covers a variety of topics that seem to get overlooked when considering the complex variables of substance abuse and ways to recover. This is a helpful read for professionals who are on the front lines of the substance abuse crisis."

Cedric Williams, Ph.D., *licensed clinical*
and consulting psychologist

Culturally Responsive Substance Use Treatment

A Guide for Practitioners, Students, and Organizations

Gabrielle Jones, Ph.D.

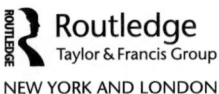

Routledge
Taylor & Francis Group

NEW YORK AND LONDON

Designed cover image: © Juliet Ekinaka – Lunations, Inc

First published 2024
by Routledge
605 Third Avenue, New York, NY 10158

and by Routledge
4 Park Square, Milton Park, Abingdon, Oxon, OX14 4RN

Routledge is an imprint of the Taylor & Francis Group, an informa business

© 2024 Gabrielle Jones

ISBN: 978-1-032-70880-5 (hbk)
ISBN: 978-1-032-70879-9 (pbk)
ISBN: 978-1-032-70882-9 (ebk)

DOI: 10.4324/9781032708829

Typeset in Times New Roman
by MPS Limited, Dehradun

To my biggest support, my most honest critic, my best friend, and husband, David. I can't imagine life without you. Thank you for your belief in my vision and your unwavering love. This book would not exist without you. I love you.

Contents

Acknowledgments

I want first to acknowledge my faith. I am grateful and humbled to have an opportunity to contribute to the larger purpose of dismantling systemically oppressive practices. Everyone deserves to be seen and everyone deserves equitable treatment. It is my hope that this book will contribute to more equity in the substance use profession beyond looking at minoritized and marginalized individuals from a deficit-focused lens.

Thank you to my family. Thank you to my mother for doing her best as a single parent and seeing that my intellect needed to be fostered. Thank you to my grandparents for being there to help raise me and instill core values of authenticity, dedication, and commitment. Thank you to my mother-in-law, late father-in-law, and sister-in-law for embracing me as family and cheering me on throughout my professional career.

I want to acknowledge the organization that raised me professionally, The Association of Black Psychologists (ABPsi). It is because of my involvement and leadership in ABPsi that I was not only able to see the injustices, but also actively work toward challenging oppressive systems, ideas, and discriminatory practices. My ABPsi family are my grounding community, and we will continue to go far together.

A heartfelt thank you to my peer-mentors, mentors, and friends who have challenged me to let my voice be heard. To my colleagues and former professors who spoke of me in rooms which I was not present and who saw something in me that I had yet to see myself, I thank you. It is because of your belief in me that I am here and will continue to engage in this much-needed multifaceted work.

Finally, I want to acknowledge those whose shoulders I stand on. The Black psychologists who blazed their own paths and created a template for my generation to follow. Thank you for showing me that there is more than one way to get to a solution and multiple ways can be correct. Thank you for showing me how to stand up for what I know is right, regardless of what people may say because they are haters and can't get beyond themselves to see the bigger picture. Thank you for speaking life and power into me when I didn't know I had it myself. Most importantly, thank you for showing me what it looks like to make real systemic change against all odds.

This book is for those who know it is time for a change. It is time to do something different because the definition of insanity is doing the same thing over and over and expecting different results.

Chapter 1

The "Why"

Culture is an ever-evolving process that involves changing, growing, and learning. Culture is not stagnant, and it looks different for different people. When I think of culture I think of generational change. I think of identities. I think of the internal belief one has of oneself that is influenced by society. When I think of culture in the context of mental health and mental health treatment, I think of the historical harm that has been inflicted on marginalized communities, the sameness of mental health treatment delivery, and how far behind the profession is regarding cultural responsiveness. The challenge that is not often discussed, and further, not translated to treatment, is the evolutionary nature of mental health. The concept of mental health often resides with evidence-based practices, but there is not often a question of who represented the population for which these evidence-based practices were developed and normed. In some cases, evidence-based practices are adapted for marginalized and minoritized groups, but the limitations remain: treatment efficacy is compared to "non-Hispanic White" populations. The evolution of culture is also impacted by things outside of our control. Natural disasters, political climate, racial epidemics, and worldwide pandemics inform culture shifts in ways we could not have imagined. An example of a once-in-a-lifetime culture shift in this generation is COVID-19. The worldwide pandemic and the abrupt changes that have occurred because of it exposed the mental health profession's severe lack of equitable treatment for marginalized and minoritized communities like one exposes a termite infestation behind rotted wood. The inequities have been there for decades, they just have not been exposed quite as starkly as they were when the world was shut down.

When developing the concept for this book, I first considered my direct care experiences. I frequently had clients of varying identities tell me how the system was not made to support them. Clients shared that they refused to go back to a residential facility for treatment due to how frequently they were misgendered, dead-named, or not considered when assigning sleeping arrangements. Parents with adolescents who used

DOI: 10.4324/9781032708829-1

substances would be crying in my office because their child was suspended or expelled for having drugs on campus that were given to them by a White student known for selling drugs on campus. They grappled with the concept that their child was suspended but the other child did not incur any consequences. Emerging adults would share that the generation of professionals providing the treatment "don't get it" and would explain that this lack of understanding is what contributed to their lack of commitment to treatment. During staff meetings, I would listen to colleagues argue over the concept of harm reduction versus abstinence, and use pejoratives to describe clients on their caseloads. Often, I found myself wondering if my colleagues really understood the history of substance use treatment and the inequities minoritized individuals faced decade after decade in substance use treatment settings. Some would argue that a book about substance use history is not helpful but rather, a book with a new cultural framework would be more beneficial. This perspective highlights the lack of understanding about how to effectively practice cultural responsiveness. A thorough understanding of *why* current substance use treatment practices are inequitable and lack cultural responsiveness is what prevents making the same mistakes in the future. This book will provide a comprehensive history of inequities as they pertain to substance use treatment and will integrate practical ways to change these traditional practices, so they are more equitable and culturally responsive. Approaches to cultural responsiveness are seamlessly woven throughout each chapter, providing the reader with historical knowledge, as well as the rationale for engaging in treatment differently. Culturally responsive substance use treatment is more than a framework, it is a fundamental shift in the way we understand substance use overall. Each chapter will provide clarity on why we need to think differently about substance use treatment to keep from repeating historical mistakes.

My professional experiences outlined above are not the only reason this book is important. The National Institute on Alcohol Abuse and Alcoholism (NIAAA), National Institute on Drug Abuse (NIDA), and Substance Abuse and Mental Health Services Administration (SAMHSA) all have names that perpetuate stigma around substance use treatment. These names are expected to be changed to reduce stigma and provide a more accurate description of their services in 2023 (APA, August 2022). The new titles proposed are the National Institute on Alcohol Effects and Alcohol-Related Disorders (formerly NIAAA), the National Institute on Drugs and Addiction (NIDA), and the Substance Use and Mental Health Services Administration (formerly SAMHSA). However, these entities have been operating under the same names for generations. The agencies leading the charge on prioritizing equity in substance use treatment have inadvertently maintained the stigma of substance use and substance use treatment. That is a huge problem! Additionally, The Mental Health Parity and Addiction Equity Act of 2008 (MHPAEA "Parity Law") required health plans and insurers that offer coverage for mental health conditions or substance use disorders to make these benefits comparable to those offered for medical and surgical benefits (Centers for Medicare & Medicaid Services, 2023). However, it was only in the 2022 Biden administration's spending bill that eliminated the "X waiver" requirement, which was a waiver that clinicians needed to obtain to provide medication-assisted treatments such as buprenorphine, which is an FDA-approved medication for Opioid Use Disorder treatment. This "X waiver" can be described as a barrier to treatment. There is no such barrier for highly addictive medications used to treat general mental health conditions such as ADHD, Depression, or Anxiety. These examples highlight how far behind substance use treatment equity is in comparison to mental health treatment.

As a licensed psychologist, it is my ethical responsibility to ensure quality and equitable mental health services are provided in my work. I found it increasingly challenging to maintain this ethical responsibility within the confines of my employers. My clients shared their experiences with other providers and the reasons they did not want to return to treatment. "My therapist called the police because I told her I wasn't going to group today. I don't know why she thought I was suicidal, I told her I wasn't. I was just angry," "I keep telling my therapist that I do not want to talk about my gender with my parents yet, but he just doesn't understand," "My entire family smokes weed, and my psychiatrist said he won't give me anything for my ADHD until I have a clean test."

The mental health industry has struggled with being equitable since the days of Sigmund Freud, commonly referred to as the "father of psychology." The American Psychological Association released a public apology in 2021 for the profession's hand in perpetuating racist practices in research and training (APA, October 2021). This apology includes a chronology of research and clinical practices dating from 1869 to the present, which contributed to harm to communities of color and to racism in America. Therapists are increasingly being faced with difficult truths but have very few solutions to the problems. The promising aspect of the mental health profession though, is that these problems are finally part of the conversation and no longer are being swept under the rug or ignored. Unfortunately, though there is progress in the mental health industry to achieve equity, substance use treatment is still heavily stigmatized. For example, substance use treatment has only recently become accessible to providers within patient records. The words we use to describe people with mental health conditions emphasize the person first. The argument made for the need for mental health treatment is that "mental health is a health issue." Clinicians across the nation are putting pen to paper and explaining to the world why seeking therapy should be akin to getting a regular physical exam. Additionally, the worldwide pandemic in 2020 shed significant light on how important mental health and well-being are to one's life expectancy and quality. Meanwhile, substance use is sort of "thrown in" as an afterthought, if at all.

Additionally, professionals in various settings are not aware of or do not feel adequately trained to fulfill their potential role in substance use care (Burrow-Sánchez et al., 2020). Clinicians in training report little to no preparation from their master's and doctorate programs as it pertains to the assessment or intervention of substance use treatment. Although this gap in training is well documented, approaches to rectify this gap are few and far between. This further highlights the disparity between mental health treatment and substance use treatment. Furthermore, the terms "cultural responsiveness," "cultural awareness," and "cultural competence" are often used but rarely defined consistently. Research has also shown the lack of cultural responsiveness in health-care and mental health treatment plays a significant role in health disparities among minoritized populations (Stubbe, 2020). Several researchers have conducted studies and literature reviews to show the significant disparities in substance use treatment among minoritized populations, identifying racism, stigma, and bias as negatively impacting quality of care for minoritized communities seeking treatment for their substance use (Lee et al., 2021; D'Amico et al., 2023). Understanding the disparities and cultural barriers to equitable treatment are crucial if progress is going to be made in equitable treatment for mental health overall, but more specifically for substance use treatment. Culturally responsive substance use looks at the individual and the people around them. Principals, program managers, coaches, and spiritual leaders all have a hand in substance use care when approaching from a culturally responsive lens.

Executives, leaders, and program managers all ask the same question. Why am I not meeting the needs of these populations? Why am I not seeing these populations in treatment programs? And what do I need to do to get people into treatment who really need it? The unfortunate thing though, is that a lot of these agencies are afraid or feel overwhelmed with what might need to happen to provide culturally responsive substance use treatment. This book is for those people. It's for leaders in organizations that actually want to provide culturally responsive substance use care by first developing a good understanding of what it means and shifting their perspectives so that they can then lead in a culturally responsive way. I worked in community mental health, I worked in hospital settings. I worked in PHP and IOP levels of care. I engaged with and collaborated with residential treatment centers and in every space, I saw a lack of culturally responsive care. I saw people being invalidated. I saw clinicians placing assumptions on minoritized individuals seeking treatment. I saw "trauma-informed care" being used without cultural considerations being addressed. I saw evidence-based treatment being used as the gold standard for care, but the populations on which the evidence was based were predominantly White. I did not see anywhere where there was a population-specific approach or group-specific approach to substance use treatment that considered cultural or identity differences. I saw people who sought treatment for substance use all being treated the same way. Their identities were ignored or minimized to create community, but instead, it was just isolating those folx who didn't feel a sense of community due to cultural differences. I saw those people leave treatment early.

As you read this book, I encourage you to take a humble posture. It is not to criticize you or your work, it is intended to give you a fresh perspective on what it truly means to provide culturally responsive substance use treatment from the inside out. Whether you are an addiction medicine expert or a mental health provider who has no idea where to start when it comes to providing equitable substance use treatment, you will develop an understanding of substance use history from a cultural perspective. You will have opportunities to explore your own biases and challenge assumptions through vignettes and case examples. Reading this book will give you practical strategies in every chapter to shift your mindset in a way that not only improves your ability to think from a culturally responsive posture as it pertains to substance use treatment but also from the way you understand and view the world. This book is intended to challenge the narrative of substance use treatment and expose the false truths that have been perpetuated through media and society. It will make you think, encourage you to take action, and provide you with hope for the future of substance use treatment.

This book was written for professionals who are committed to making a change but don't know where to start. It is for the therapist who hesitates to take on a client with a substance use issue. This book is for the organizations that struggle to get minoritized communities in the door to access their services. For far too long, substance use treatment has been inconsistent, unclear, and taboo. It is time to change the narrative and that starts by developing a conceptual framework and understanding of what culturally responsive substance use treatment means, what it looks like, and practical ways to engage in such treatment. It is my hope that when you finish this book, you feel enlightened, empowered, and encouraged to adapt your practices to look more culturally responsive for substance use treatment, and for mental health treatment overall.

You will notice throughout the book that the term "field" is not used, but instead, you will see "profession" or "industry." Language is important when we are discussing cultural responsiveness and just as saying "I am sitting Indian style" can be offensive to Indigenous communities, the term "field" can be seen as insensitive to individuals historically forced to do work in a "field," minimizing how challenging that type of work is in comparison. Other phrases you will notice include "marginalized and minoritized individuals." These phrases highlight the societal influence placed on individuals from varying ethnic and racial backgrounds. People of varying ethnic and racial backgrounds are people first, and society has marginalized and minoritized people to create power differentials and institutionalized oppression. The effort to use different language to discuss diversity more accurately and appropriately is an important part of this book. Finally, you will note that person-first language is used throughout the book. This was done to reduce stigma by reinforcing culturally responsive practices in the development of this book. As mentioned, culture is ever-evolving, and as such, some phrases and terms will undoubtedly be deemed culturally insensitive at some point. Please keep this in mind as you read and recognize that, while attempts are made to be culturally responsive in every way, human error is inevitable. If you are reading this book, I encourage you to give yourself grace in this area as well and be open and willing to learn and evolve with culture.

References

American Psychological Association. (2021, October 29). APA apologizes for longstanding contributions to systemic racism [Press release]. https://www.apa.org/news/press/releases/2021/10/apology-systemic-racism

American Psychological Association. (2022, August 17). Names of addiction-related federal agencies are changing. https://www.apaservices.org/advocacy/news/addiction-related-federal-agencies

Burrow-Sánchez, J. J., Martin, J. L., & Taylor, J. M. (2020). The need for training psychologists in substance use disorders. *Training and Education in Professional Psychology*, *14*(1), 8–18. 10.1037/tep0000262

Centers for Medicare & Medicaid Services. (2023, September 6). Mental health parity & addiction equity act (MHPAEA). Centers for Medicare & Medicaid Services. https://www.cms.gov/marketplace/private-health-insurance/mental-health-parity-addiction-equity

D'Amico, E. J., Tucker, J. S., Dunbar, M. S., Perez, L., Siconolfi, D., Davis, J. P., Pedersen, E. R., & Rodriguez, A. (2023). Unpacking disparities in substance-related outcomes among racial, ethnic, sexual, and gender minoritized groups during adolescence and emerging adulthood. *Psychology of Addictive Behaviors*, *37*(5), 651–656. 10.1037/adb0000905

Lee, C. S., O'Connor, B. M., Todorova, I., Nicholls, M. E., & Colby, S. M. (2021). Structural racism and reflections from Latinx heavy drinkers: Impact on mental health and alcohol use. *Journal of Substance Abuse Treatment*, *127*, 108352. 10.1016/j.jsat.2021.108352

Stubbe, D. E. (2020, January 24). Practicing cultural competence and cultural humility in the care of diverse patients. *Journal of Lifelong Learning in Psychiatry*, *18*(1), 49–51. 10.1176/appi.focus.20190041

Chapter 2

Substance Use

The "Moral Issue"

Mental health concerns vary widely among humanity. However, there are some mental health issues that clinicians will not touch with a 10-foot pole. Disordered eating? Yikes. Schizophrenia? No thanks. Harm OCD? Hard pass.

Some clinicians are extremely passionate about these diagnoses, have designated expertise in these areas, and provide valuable services to these communities. Nonetheless, when it comes to substance use, there tend to be fewer clinicians ready and willing to provide care (Priester et al., 2016). One reason for this is that clinicians do not receive adequate training in this area and as a result do not feel equipped to provide substance use treatment (Burrow-Sánchez et al., 2020), but that can also be said for diagnoses such as disordered eating, schizophrenia, and Harm OCD. Additionally, substance use is heavily stigmatized, which contributes to lack of screening or assessment of substance use by non-specialized providers (Van Boekel et al., 2013; Yang et al., 2017). Still, the same can be said for the first three diagnoses listed. This brings me to the reason I think many clinicians hit pause when they are asked to do substance use treatment.

It's STILL treated as a moral issue.

This chapter will provide a detailed overview of the way substance use was conceptualized from the 1600s on, beginning with the thought that alcohol addiction was primarily due to immorality. In this chapter, you will also see the transition from alcohol use being "immoral" to it being seen as an incurable disease, to a maladaptive behavior. This trajectory will culminate in the current conceptualization of substance use, in general, being seen as a combination of disease, morality, and maladaptive behavior. The inconsistencies and lack of agreement among professionals highlights the current stigma associated with substance use.

I will also discuss how substance use is depicted today through various platforms. Social media, commercials, and movies have always played a

DOI: 10.4324/9781032708829-2

key role in how substance use is accepted or rejected within communities. These outlets have also contributed to the cultural substance use biases that are developed and held by society. Raising awareness of how substance use has been depicted from a social context will help you develop a clear understanding of how society thinks about substances and substance use from a culturally informed angle. Raising awareness of this nuanced intersection of culture and substance use perception is a necessary component to reduce stigma and change the narrative placed on people who use substances. Understanding the societal influences on one's interpretation of substance use emphasizes the racial overtones placed on the use of certain substances, which is often what leaks into our subconscious and contributes to how vastly different certain substances are treated depending on who is seen using them. Additionally, this chapter focuses on social media, commercials, and movie depictions of substance use, ranging from a "good time" to "the worst night ever," outlining how mixed the perception of substance use is within our society. In this chapter, you will also find discussion related to providers' level of discomfort working with people who engage in substance use, and how the lack of consistency among professionals about the root cause of substance use contributes to this discomfort.

History of Substance Use Conceptualization

When discussing substance use history, most books start with discussing alcohol use because it was a unifying beverage for Americans dating back to the 1600s. Alcohol's history is not much different from what we see in other substance stories. It started out as a magic cure, a joyful elixir with no harmful risks of use. Alcohol, when consumed in excess at the time, was regarded as no more than an annoyance. Consider your family holidays. Do you have that one uncle or cousin who everyone sees as a nuisance? "Oh, that's just Uncle Mike, he's harmless!!" Well, alcohol was "Uncle Mike" in the 1600s. Americans dismissed alcohol overuse as a character flaw and thought nothing more of it. Anyone who ended up sick was sick because of their own moral flaws. Overconsumption was a choice.

However, the medical profession came to realize that there were more factors contributing to alcohol use; more medical issues that were incurable. This perspective shift for alcohol started in the late 1700s through the book, "The Diseases of Workers," in which the author, Swedish physician Magnus Huss, utilized "alcoholism" as a medical term to describe individuals who have used alcohol in excess and developed medical conditions as a result. As it turns out, Uncle Mike was NOT harmless after all. Even during the prohibition era of the 1920s "medicinal alcohol" was exempt. It was not until Alcoholics Anonymous (AA), founded in 1935, though, that the medical model of addiction became mainstream. One of the two AA founders, "Dr. Bob" as he was affectionately called, is who really validated the "disease model" of addiction due to his own personal experience with severe alcohol use. Because he had a medical degree, and because *he* was not able to truly recover from his addiction, his perception was that no one could. This idea was the very foundation of the disease model and was very lucrative for the medical industry. By 1980, it was well established that alcohol addiction was an incurable medical condition, making its way into the DSM-III and eventually branching out in subsequent DSMs to be one of many substance use disorders. Since then, the medical profession continued to develop a framework to conceptualize substance use disorders. Behaviorists provided their conceptualization of addiction as a learned behavior, and psychoanalysts provided their conceptualization of addiction as the result of childhood trauma or unmet needs. Throughout history, the medical profession has made attempts to adapt the definition of addiction. A key example is the American Society of Addiction Medicine's (ASAM) evolution of the definition of addiction (ASAM, n.d.):

1991: primary, chronic disease of brain reward, motivation, memory, and related circuitry.

2011: primary, chronic disease of brain reward, motivation, memory, and related circuitry. Dysfunction in these circuits leads to characteristic biological, psychological, social, and spiritual manifestations. This is reflected in an individual pathologically pursuing reward and/or relief by substance use and other behaviors.

2019: treatable, chronic medical disease involving complex interactions among brain circuits, genetics, the environment, and an individual's life experiences. People with addiction use substances or engage in behaviors that become compulsive and often continue despite harmful consequences. Prevention efforts and treatment approaches for addiction are generally as successful as those for other chronic diseases.

Though these are not every iteration of the addiction definition, these definitions reflect the progression of how alcohol use was conceptualized over the years. The current definition of addiction released by ASAM acknowledges the treatable nature of substance use and attempts to incorporate the biological, psychological, and social aspects of addiction. It also acknowledges that prevention and treatment are effective. You would think, since this definition is more comprehensive and inclusive, that there would be cohesion among providers, but there is not. Providers still disagree on the origin of one's substance use, and as such, develop contrasting treatment interventions. Unfortunately, the lack of cohesion harms people who use substances the most.

Stigma

Several articles debunk the archaic perspective that substance use is a moral issue (Frank & Nagel, 2017; Thombs & Osborn, 2019). However, one conflict that continues to make people think having a substance use disorder is a moral issue is the categorization of substance use. Substance use categorization means some people are labeled "social drinkers" while others are labeled "binge drinkers." Some people are labeled "problem drinkers" and finally we have people who have been diagnosed with full blown alcohol use disorders. This idea of categorization also spans to type of substance. People who use cocaine or heroin are not categorized as "social cocaine users" or "social heroin users." Additionally, people who have prescription substance use challenges are generally categorized as having a "tissue-dependence" contributing to their prescription medication addiction. Having an addiction to prescription medication is the only addiction that our culture fully embraces as a medical condition. Wonder why? This will be addressed in later chapters. When discussing people who use cannabis, some are labeled as "potheads" with no categorization associated with how much of the substance is being consumed. Someone who uses cannabis can smoke or vape on occasion, use daily, or dab, vape, and ingest edibles in the same day; each of those people can still be labeled a "pothead."

These varying forms of substance use categorization reinforce the strength of the moral argument. The lack of consistency in what constitutes addiction depending on the substance, the subjective nature of labeling who does what substance, and the social taboo related to certain substances make it very challenging for people to break their association with substance use having more to do with one's lack of control than one's substance use being understood as a medical condition. The DSM-5TR and DSMs prior have attempted to stan-dardize what constitutes an addiction, namely by identifying that there is "clinically significant impairment or distress" resulting from the pattern of use. Unfortunately, this is very subjective to the client and the therapist, and often does not account for cultural stressors that may compound clinically significant distress (Lee et al., 2013). This qualifier also may not be an issue for someone who uses prescription medications in excess and does not experience clinically significant impairment or distress. When placing these concepts on other diagnoses such as OCD or schizophrenia, there is not a categorization comparison. The social component of one's OCD behavior isn't labeled as "social," in contrast the diagnosis of OCD is often overgeneralized to people who simply like a clean home, or those who do not like clutter. In some cases, the OCD "label" represents a point of pride. Some people say, "it's just my OCD" and that is accepted. The same cannot be said for substance use. The desire to reduce clutter does not hinder one's daily life, nor does the *lack* of a clean home or *having* clutter cause them significant clinical distress. This leads to the following questions: If there are social drinkers who can stop whenever they want, how come people with alcohol use disorder can't? If someone is diagnosed with a mild alcohol use disorder, does that mean they *can* stop?

In the substance use world, anyone who can or does use socially but does not have an addiction is affectionately called a "normy." It is most common when referring to people who drink alcohol by people who do not drink alcohol because of their alcohol use disorder. This "nick-name" is used to insinuate that people who are not able to drink or engage in substance use socially are "normal" and everyone else is damaged or has a problem. This is the foundation of substance use stigma. The idea that someone who has a substance use disorder is not normal, or someone who uses substances "socially" *is* normal is extremely problematic. Conversely, people who are in recovery from their substance use call themselves "addicts." This is particularly common in recovery meetings. They say their name and declare their addiction to substances. This process over decades has created an identity. The statement, "I am an addict," has become a point of pride for some, as it represents not only who they believe they are, but also an admission of their past transgressions and the idea that addiction is forever their identity. What many fail to realize is this declaration of addiction has the capacity to ignore all other aspects of a person's identity. It also reinforces the moral flaw conceptualization of substance use and increases stigma of substance use disorders. The 'addict' label can elicit shame, guilt, or blame if used to describe someone in recovery. In the general mental health discussion, there is much encouragement to use person-first language, that is, refer to the person, then identify the behavior in which they engage. An example of this would be, "person with anxiety." If this concept is used for addiction, the example would be "person with a substance use disorder," or "person who uses substances." This form of describing someone who uses substances helps remove the label of "addict" and opens the door for the person who uses substances to understand that their substance use does not have to be who they are; it doesn't have to define them. They have an opportunity to learn about what aspects of themselves they would like to focus on. Using person-first language not only reduces substance use stigma, it also provides individuals a chance to see themselves beyond their addiction or substance use.

Society's Depiction of Substance Use

Early sociological theories, such as the theory of social control, define societal behavior as being informed by social norms (Janowitz, 1975). More recently, studies have shown that when someone does a kind act, others are more inclined to express gratitude and experience higher life satisfaction (Datu et al., 2022). If people are more prone to have a grateful posture after simply observing acts of kindness from others, it can be deduced that people can develop more favorable perceptions of substance use if it is depicted positively. Alternatively, if people are exposed to more negative depictions of substance use, a more negative perception is adopted. A cultural example of how media has contributed to social perception is the show *Will & Grace*.

Will & Grace was an American sitcom that first debuted on air in 1998 and ran until 2006. This period coincided with efforts to increase gender equality through legalization of same-sex marriage, which gained traction in the 1990s and finally succeeded through supreme court judgement in 2015. The show followed the lives of two best friends, Will Truman (a self-identified gay lawyer) and Grace Adler (a self-identified straight interior designer), along with their eccentric friends, Karen Walker and Jack McFarland. Through its comedy and relatable characters, *Will & Grace* played a key role in positively impacting society's comfort with same-sex marriage and LGBTQIA+ rights.

One of the significant ways the show impacted societal perception was through its portrayal of individuals from the LGBTQIA+ community. At a time when representation of LGBTQIA+ individuals was limited on television, *Will & Grace* introduced a gay lead character, Will Truman, who was depicted as a successful, intelligent, and relatable individual. Will's character helped break stereotypes and humanize gay men on television, showing that their lives were not defined solely by their sexual orientation. The show also addressed social issues such as coming out, relationships, and gay rights in a comedic and approachable manner. It tackled important subjects with humor, using its platform to raise awareness and generate discussion within social circles. By presenting individuals from the LGBTQIA+ community as part of everyday life, the show helped to normalize same-sex relationships and showcased the challenges and joys experienced by the LGBTQIA+ community.

The dynamic friendship between Will and Grace, regardless of their different sexual orientations, demonstrated that LGBTQIA+ individuals can have deep and meaningful connections with their straight counterparts. The show emphasized the importance of acceptance, understanding, and love between friends, whatever their sexual orientation. This portrayal helped break down barriers and fostered empathy and support for the

LGBTQIA+ community in society. *Will & Grace* also played a significant role in the push for same-sex marriage acceptance. The show often depicted the struggles faced by Will and his romantic partners, highlighting the inequities and challenges they encountered due to the lack of legal recognition for same-sex relationships. By presenting these narratives, the show contributed to the broader conversation on marriage equality and helped shape public opinion.

Moreover, the cultural impact of *Will & Grace* extended beyond its TV viewership. The show was widely discussed and referenced in popular culture, making its characters and storylines accessible to a broad audience. The visibility and positive representation of individuals from the LGBTQIA+ community on such a mainstream platform helped challenge prejudices and stereotypes carried by individuals in society and allowed for a more nuanced understanding of the LGBTQIA+ community. Overall, *Will & Grace* had a substantial positive impact on society's comfort with same-sex marriage and LGBTQIA+ rights. By normalizing LGBTQIA+ characters and relationships, the show helped reduce stigma, increase acceptance, and promote equality. It showcased the power of media in shaping societal perceptions, paving the way for greater understanding and support for the LGBTQIA+ community.

Herein lies why discussing society's depiction of substance use is integral in understanding what culturally responsive substance use treatment means. As a professional, it is critical to be able to see the proverbial forest from the trees when viewing depictions of people who use heroin and people who use cannabis. These images and depictions are not necessarily accurate and can actually be harmful by increasing biases and prejudices about people who use certain substances. These individuals are shown in a way that society has adopted through media outlets to elicit emotional responses. Like the show *Will & Grace*, many television shows that are based on substance use have the power to influence our culture in meaningful ways. *Will & Grace* as a show was intentional regarding the exploration of differences and the nuances of living in a world that did not respect or appreciate those differences at the time it was being aired. It is important to recognize how much media influence plays a role in how we as providers perceive someone who uses a particular substance. Recognizing the potential biases developed from common media platforms is a step toward increasing cultural awareness.

Ads are a consistent example of how society can be influenced based on what is seen. People who develop ad campaigns study what type of images contribute to an increase in consumer purchases. Great attention is given to the look of a person in an ad and what content is presented in an ad. Take cigarette ads for example: The image of a thin White woman, seductively looking over her shoulder with an "Old Gold" brand cigarette in her hand, and the tagline "Straight from the shoulder ... If you want a treat instead of a treatment ... smoke Old Golds" is intended to elicit an emotional reaction. There are no infographics or nutrition facts on the ad, just the woman, the cigarettes, and the words. People respond positively due to the positive depiction, and women smoking Old Golds becomes a social norm. However, this representation may not match the person you see coming through treatment doors. The perception that providers have of what type of person enters substance use treatment can also contribute to the severe lack of access to treatment among minoritized individuals. According to a recent publication from the Yale school of medicine, 90% of Black Americans and 92% of Latinx individuals who were diagnosed with a substance use disorder did not receive addiction treatment (Cruz, 2021). The research is clear that racism and institutionalized practices play a role in this disparity, but we also need to consider the covert nature of media's contribution to these biases, which also contribute to these disparities.

The way in which society has informed and influenced the perception of people who use substances can be understood through social media, commercials, television shows, and movies. It is important to also note that as society changes in other ways, such as through technology or a global pandemic, so does society's depiction of people who use substances.

Social Media

Social media has evolved at warp speed over the past twenty years and continues to evolve more rapidly as technology becomes more advanced. Technology has made significant advancements from staying connected to friends and family across the globe to having a video for DIY patio installment at your fingertips. The advancements have created a world where social media is at the forefront of fashion trends, academic information, and professional presence. These innovative forms of communication have also exposed significant inequities among minoritized populations. Social media is where we go to see the latest updates about recent police shootings of unarmed Black people. Social media is the place we may discover another senseless and tragic mass shooting in a LGBTQIA+ space. We use social media to challenge oppression and injustices through #StopAsianHate #MeToo and #BlackLivesMatter hashtags. In most of these social media examples, there are two sides: those who are in support, and those who oppose.

Unfortunately, the same cannot be said for substance use or substance use treatment. The lack of consistency in social media regarding substance use creates biases and harmful narratives regarding how people perceive substance use. Consider these two social media examples when thinking about how social media can influence social norms around substance use.

Example 1: A "BORG" (Blackout Rage Gallon), is a plastic gallon jug filled with a combination of water, alcohol, flavoring, and electrolytes. Some of these "BORGs" may also contain caffeine. BORGs were introduced on the social media platform TikTok, in which many college students were conducting tutorials about how to make them. The concept started trending instantly and many White college students who are considered "Gen Z" adopted the idea of bringing BORGs to parties with them. Quickly, a set of substance use providers presented the concept as a harm-reduction strategy. The perception of bringing your own alcohol to binge drink was positive. The providers argued that this approach to college drinking is safer than drinking whatever is at a party because (1) the students know what is in their drink, (2) there is a finite amount, reducing the likelihood that one would overconsume, and (3) the concoction is mixed with water, reducing the likelihood that someone would become dehydrated when drinking. Think about how the response may have looked differently if the BORGs were introduced by Black students.

Example 2: In 2021, a woman named Sha'Carri Richardson secured a spot on the U.S. Olympic track and field team after winning the women's 100-meter race in the Olympic trials. She was seen as an inspiration for young Black girls and she was rapidly gaining attention for her talent. Sha'Carri was informed that her biological mother unexpectedly passed away a few days following her win in the Olympic trials. She consumed marijuana to cope with this challenging and unexpected news, and because marijuana was in her system, her Olympic team position was rescinded, and she was not able to compete in the Tokyo Olympics. Quickly, social media content became saturated with attacks on Sha'Carri's character, insults about her physical appearance, and criticism of her behavior. Within a few months of this situation, another Olympic competitor, 15-year-old Russian figure skater, Kamila Valieva, had a detected drug test for a substance considered to function as a stimulant in the Olympics (Trimetazidine). This substance is listed on the World Anti-Doping Agency list for substances that constitute a ban from Olympic participation. However, social media came to Kamila's defense, arguing that not allowing her to participate would contribute to emotional harm. No attacks on her character, no insults, and no criticism came from this situation, yet the substance detected is explicitly labeled as a performance enhancement. The illustration here is not to argue whether using substances is correct or incorrect, instead, it is to show explicitly how different responses via social media to substance use are rooted in bias and prejudice.

Consider these examples when thinking about how social media can impact society's perception of a substance, the "types" of people who use it, and its "positive or negative" depictions.

Commercials

Although many streaming services provide the option of commercial-free viewing, commercial advertisements still manage to make their way into society's cognition when assessing substance use. One of the most iconic commercials of the early 2000s was Budweiser's "whassup" commercial, in which several people called each other while drinking their beer, saying "whassup." This commercial developed into a worldwide phenomenon, crossing several cultural barriers, and creating a communal identity. There are many non-substance related commercials that have increased consumer purchasing of the product and promote brand awareness, but the key issue to be pointed out with commercials is what gets commercialized and what does not.

Consider this: alcohol commercials have been consistent and generally positive. Even if alcohol is not being promoted, the social situation in the commercial may be evening cocktails or drinks with friends. These commercials are almost always positive, creating an ideal that consumers want to make reality, and these commercials are almost always cast with adults. Alternatively, we see commercials with vaping that are geared toward prevention or abstinence. These commercials often cast adolescents and are promoted through a drug-free type of campaign. Alternatively, there are very few commercials with people engaging in cocaine, heroin, or prescription substance use. If we do see those commercials, they are intended to make a lasting impact that encourages people to seek professional help. How do you feel after reading through these commercial examples? Consider the biases you carry and how commercials have influenced your perception about substance use and those who use certain substances.

Alcohol overconsumption contributes to 3 million deaths per year, which is 5.3% of all deaths according to the World Health Organization (WHO, 2018). This means alcohol-related deaths are the third leading risk factor for premature death and disability worldwide! High blood pressure and tobacco use are numbers one and two respectively. If alcohol is the third leading risk factor for premature death only behind high blood pressure and tobacco use, why do most of our substance related commercials promote drinking behaviors? Why are policies and regulations focused on controlling cannabis? Society does not see alcohol as a health issue, nor does our society want to see alcohol as a health risk. Content in commercials and the way certain substances are depicted contribute to this lack of concern for alcohol and heightened concern for other substances.

Movies

Movies are where writers, directors, producers, and actors come together to reflect accurate or exaggerated aspects of the world in which we live. Often you will glean rich artistic expressions when watching movies. Movies also play a significant role in shaping society's perception of substance use and substance use treatment. Although social media and commercials have the capacity to elicit strong emotions and facilitate connection among different identities, movies can accomplish this while also taking you on a journey. From character development to setting, movies give you an opportunity to become invested in the story, not just the product. The amount of investment put into movies is transferred to those who watch, and this is why I would argue that movies are *most* influential in the development of society's perception of who uses certain substances, which substances are "bad," and substance use treatment stigma.

Because movies are released constantly and the substance use world is ever changing, it is important to keep in mind the larger intention behind examples provided. The intention is to encourage you to pay attention to how subtle opinions and inferences develop due to how substance use and substance use treatment are depicted in movies.

In November 2015, a movie called *The Night Before* was released. This movie was about three friends who grew up together and supported each other through one friend's unexpected loss of his parents. The three friends commit to spending every Christmas Eve together so the newly orphaned friend would never be alone. The movie carries this tradition through the lives of the three friends as they grow into adulthood and develop lives of their own. One friend has a celebrity lifestyle, one friend has a family and is expecting his first child, and the orphaned friend is struggling with transitioning into adulthood. Roughly 15 years into their Christmas Eve tradition, the two supportive friends agree that this tradition needs to end. They recognize they cannot engage in the same behaviors they did when they were younger. The last "hoorah" of the tradition includes the use of several substances and a few comedic substance related mishaps. Though this movie is heavily influenced by substance use, the story within it is where people identify. The tragedies of life, ebbs and flows of friendship, and transitioning into adulthood are all non-discriminatory aspects of this movie. The depiction of how substances affect the characters, though, puts forth a perception of specific substances. Throughout the movie, when characters have alcohol, there are no mishaps. However, when characters smoke cannabis, there are mishaps. These minor artistic choices to tell the story influence how the viewer begins to perceive alcohol versus cannabis. Additionally, the movie is about friends, not drugs (explicitly) so it is easy for the audience to overlook these differences.

Raising awareness is one of the most important aspects of being able to understand what it means to engage in culturally responsive substance use treatment. Seeing the role of social media, commercials, and movies in how substance use is understood in society is helpful in more accurately contextualizing substance use.

Lack of Provider Comfort with Substance Use

Foundational psychology courses focus on the history of psychology, diagnosis in psychology, human development, and broad overviews of different psychological approaches to treatment. As providers become more specialized in mental health through graduate school, courses focus more directly on assessment, conceptualization, and intervention approaches to diagnoses. Specialization in a specific diagnosis expertise, for example, eating disorders, psychotic disorders, or substance use disorders, comes more from the interest of the trainee and clinical experience. If you are interested in developing expertise in disordered eating behavior, you would choose the elective or continuing education courses to obtain that knowledge. This can be said for most subject matter experts in the profession. Unfortunately, though, many providers elect to become subject matter experts in areas other than substance use. The lack of clinician match (that is when the clinician and client have similar cultural backgrounds) is an additional indicator that providers are not matriculating into the substance use profession (Gainsbury, 2016). Furthermore, it is well documented that there is a gap in training related to substance use treatment, leading providers to feel ill-equipped to address substance use concerns in their areas (Ram & Chisolm, 2016). Bias providers carry toward people who have been diagnosed with substance use disorder can stem from the media, as outlined in the previous section. The media depictions can also contribute to stigma and lead providers to believe harmful narratives including: people who use substances are "manipulative," or people who use substances "don't want to stop using." These perceptions coupled with lack of training, bleed into how providers approach working with people who have substance use disorders, and often contribute to lack of cultural responsiveness in treatment. Additionally, providers have an added responsibility to address medical considerations for someone who has a substance use disorder. Withdrawal, overdose, and relapse are all real and quite dangerous factors to consider in substance use treatment. Training programs rarely provide explicit education on how to manage relapse, or what to do in a situation where a client is withdrawing from a substance. Moreover, symptoms such as withdrawal do require medical attention, and many facilities do not have the resources to manage substance use withdrawal, thereby eliminating the possibility for substance use treatment all together.

As mentioned earlier in this chapter, there are several schools of thought as they pertain to a provider's conceptualization of substance use origin (White & Kurtz, 2006). A lack of agreement among providers breeds discomfort. Substance use falls in the gray area, making it more challenging or providers to feel comfortable providing treatment. Furthermore, given the strong history of AA's approach to utilizing peer support in recovery, many providers who deliver substance use treatment are themselves in recovery. This dynamic has created an unspoken barrier for providers who are not in recovery feeling as though they are not able or qualified to provide substance use treatment. In every position I have had, as a trainee and as a professional, I was asked by at least one client if I was in recovery. To this day, I have not and will not answer that question. However, on several occasions I have had group co-leaders, managers, and supervisors self-disclose to clients that they are in recovery. I do not answer this question for several reasons. First, the answer does not change my approach when working with clients. Second, the answer does not consistently provide clinical benefit and can contribute to overidentification or a therapeutic rupture between me and the client. Thirdly, I am entitled to privacy as a provider. When working with a person who has been diagnosed with a psychotic disorder, is it customary to share whether you have a psychotic disorder? What about depression?

Because the culture of substance use treatment is such that providers are generally in recovery themselves, hesitation grows when therapists are interested in obtaining expertise in substance use treatment but are not in recovery. If a therapist is not in recovery themselves and is presented with the expectation that they share their personal substance use, they are faced with a dilemma that might prevent them from developing expertise in this area. Culturally responsive substance use treatment does not require self-disclosure. It requires humility and an openness to understand another person's experience that may be different from your own. I encourage you to consider why *you* may feel uncomfortable when met with the possibility of delivering substance use treatment and see if any of these reasons resonate.

To address the inconsistencies among professionals in understanding substance use, the Biological-Psychological-Social (bio-psycho-social) model provides a comprehensive framework that acknowledges the multi-faceted nature of substance use disorders. This model highlights the intersection of biological, psychological, and social factors that interact with each other to influence an individual's level of risk for substance use, addiction, and its maintenance (Skewes & Gonzalez, 2013). The bio-psycho-social framework is one approach that takes more than genetic predisposition into consideration when conceptualizing substance use treatment and can be utilized to inform more culturally responsive interventions based on individualized bio-psycho-social influences. When looking at biological factors that contribute to addiction, this can look like genetic predispositions. An example of this would be if someone has two biological parents who have substance use disorders. Their risk of developing a substance use disorder themselves is increased because of their parent's substance use. This does not mean the person with parents who have addiction will in fact develop a substance use disorder, it simply means there is an increased risk for them compared to an individual who does not have parents with substance use disorders. Psychologically, if someone has a mental health diagnosis, anxiety disorder for example, they are more likely to develop co-occurring substance use disorder (Vorspan et al., 2015) than their counterparts who do not have a mental health diagnosis. The social component of the bio-psycho-social model can be situations in which your core social group engages in activities that primarily center on substance use. It is important to note that just because any one or all three of these aspects of one's life can be true, does not indicate that the person will develop a substance use disorder. It only increases the risk of developing a substance use disorder. With that said, developing interventions that target specific aspects of an individual's life in one or all three of these areas is an adequate start to delivering culturally responsive substance use treatment. By adopting a more holistic approach and integrating these factors into treatment, providers can also enhance their understanding and comfort in working with individuals who engage in substance use.

To address providers' discomfort and promote consistency in under-standing substance use, a multipronged approach, similar to a holistic treatment approach, is necessary. Though there is education and training available in substance use treatment, the societal stigma associated with substance use needs to be targeted. Promoting self-reflection and cultural humility, fostering collaborative and non-judgmental therapeutic relationships, and engaging in interdisciplinary collaborations are several potential starting points to begin addressing substance use stigma (Center for Behavioral Health Statistics and Quality, 2016). By engaging in any one of the practices listed above, there is also an opportunity to contribute to changing the social narrative of substance use treatment. Providing substance use treatment does not need to be everyone's answer, but increasing accurate knowledge of substance use disorders and substance use treatment can contribute to challenging biases and reducing stigma. As with any expertise, additional ongoing supervision and consultation also reduce biases and increase cultural humility when working with people who have substance use disorders.

Overall, the profession of substance use treatment is still split regarding why substance use disorders develop, and social depictions of substance use have contributed to the disparities in treatment approaches and biases toward people who use certain substances. To break these stigma barriers, it is critical to pay attention to how substance use is portrayed in the media. Using consultation and ongoing supervision to check individual biases is also important for providers to develop a deeper and more comprehensive understanding of substance use and substance use treatment. It does not require an individual to provide substance use treatment to contribute to breaking the stigma, it just takes a willingness to approach the topic humbly and with an open mind. If we can change the narrative to one that is more accurate, culturally responsive, and holistic, it is possible that more individuals can and will seek training and education to provide the much-needed culturally responsive substance use treatment to people who have substance use disorders. Further, those who need treatment will also be more likely to obtain treatment knowing that their providers are offering culturally responsive care.

References

American Society of Addiction Medicine (ASAM). (n.d.). Definition of addiction. https://www.asam.org/quality-care/definition-of-addiction

Burrow-Sánchez, J. J., Martin, J. L., & Taylor, J. M. (2020). The need for training psychologists in substance use disorders. *Training and Education in Professional Psychology, 14*(1), 8–18. 10.1037/tep0000262

Center for Behavioral Health Statistics and Quality. (2016). *2015 National Survey on Drug Use and Health: Detailed Tables. Substance Abuse and Mental Health Services Administration*. Rockville, MD.

Cruz, F. (2021). Racial inequities in treatments of addictive disorders. *American Academy of Addiction Psychiatry*. https://medicine.yale.edu/news-article/racial-inequities-in-treatments-of-addictive-disorders/

D'Amico, E. J., Tucker, J. S., Dunbar, M. S., Perez, L., Siconolfi, D., Davis, J. P., Pedersen, E. R., & Rodriguez, A. (2023). Unpacking disparities in substance-related outcomes among racial, ethnic, sexual, and gender minoritized groups during adolescence and emerging adulthood. *Psychology of Addictive Behaviors, 37*(5), 651–656. 10.1037/adb0000905

Datu, J. A. D., Valdez, J. P. M., McInerney, D. M., & Cayubit, R. F. (2022). The effects of gratitude and kindness on life satisfaction, positive emotions, negative emotions, and COVID-19 anxiety: An online pilot experimental study. *Applied Psychology. Health and Well-being, 14*(2), 347–361. 10.1111/aphw.12306

Frank, L. E., & Nagel, S. K. (2017). Addiction and moralization: The role of the underlying model of addiction. *Neuroethics, 10*(1), 129–139. 10.1007/s12152-017-9307-x

Gainsbury, S. M. (2016). Cultural competence in the treatment of addictions: Theory, practice, and evidence. *Clinical Psychology and Psychotherapy, 24*(4), 987–1001.

Janowitz, M. (1975). Sociological theory and social control. *American Journal of Sociology, 81*(1), 82–108.

Lee, C. S., Colby, S. M., Rohsenow, D. J., López, S. R., Hernández, L., & Caetano, R. (2013). Acculturation stress and drinking problems among urban heavy drinking Latinos in the Northeast. *Journal of Ethnicity in Substance Abuse, 12*(4), 308–320. 10.1080/15332640.2013.830942

Priester, M. A., Browne, T., Iachini, A., Clone, S., DeHart, D., & Seay, K. D. (2016). Treatment access barriers and disparities among individuals with co-occurring mental health and substance use disorders: An integrative literature review. *Journal of Substance Abuse Treatment, 61*, 47–59. 10.1016/j.jsat.2015.09.006

Ram, A., & Chisolm, M. S. (2016). The time is now: Improving substance abuse training in medical schools. *Academic Psychiatry: The Journal of the American Association of Directors of Psychiatric Residency Training and the Association for Academic Psychiatry, 40*(3), 454–460. 10.1007/s40596-015-0314-0

Skewes, M. C., & Gonzalez, V. M. (2013). The biopsychosocial model of addiction. In *Principles of addiction* (pp. 61–70). 10.1016/B978-0-12-398336-7.00006-1

Staff, R. (2022, January 28). Sha'Carri Richardson slams Olympics' 'hypocrisy' over doping rules: 'Just let us run'. *Rolling Stone*. https://www.rollingstone.com/culture/culture-news/shacarri-richardson-slams-olympics-doping-marijuana-1299997/

Thombs, D. L., & Osborn, C. J. (2019). *Introduction to addictive behaviors* (5th ed.). Guilford Press.

Van Boekel, L., Brouwers, E. P. M., Weeghel, J. V., & Garretsen, H. F. L. (2013). Stigma among health professionals towards patients with substance use disorders and its consequences for healthcare delivery: Systematic review. *Drug and Alcohol Dependence, 131*(1–2), 23–35. 10.1016/j.drugalcdep.2013.02.018

Vorspan, F., Mehtelli, W., Dupuy, G., Bloch, V., & Lépine, J. P. (2015). Anxiety and substance use disorders: Co-occurrence and clinical issues. *Current Psychiatry Reports, 17*, 1–7.

White, W. , & Kurtz, E. (2006). The varieties of recovery experience. *International Journal of Self Help and Self Care*, *3*(1–2), 21–61. 10.2190/911R-MTQ5-VJ1H-75CU

World Health Organization. (2018). *Global status report on alcohol and health 2018*. Retrieved from https://www.who.int/publications/i/item/9789241565639

Yang, L. H., Wong, L. Y., Grivel, M. M., & Hasin, D. S. (2017). Stigma and substance use disorders: An international phenomenon. *Current Opinion in Psychiatry*, *30*(5), 378–388. 10.1097/YCO.0000000000000351

Chapter 3

Substance Use and the Workplace

Substance use in the workplace has a complex history shaped by social, cultural, and legal factors. It has also gone through several iterations over the course of history and its perception and acceptance have varied across different times and cultures. The use of substances such as alcohol and tobacco in the workplace can be traced back to early industrial generations. It was not uncommon for employees to use substances during work to help manage the work being done. Physically taxing jobs and non-potable water also prompted significant adoption of alcohol consumption by workers (Olson & Gerstein, 1985). Opioids were introduced as prescribed medications for sustained injuries in labor intensive work environments to help manage chronic pain. They were also promoted as "non-habit-forming" or "nonaddictive" in the early 2000s when opioid prescriptions increased significantly. Unfortunately, culture played a significant role in the increase of substance use to manage harsh working conditions as many people working "blue-collar" jobs were the same people in need of relief from the toll their work took on their bodies. Unde et al. (2012) found that people with lower socioeconomic status and lower level of education were more likely to have lower back pain due to labor intensive jobs. They also found that there was a correlation between lower back pain and smoking. Furman (2012) identified stressors related to immigration for undocumented LatinX men as a contributing factor to substance use. Specifically, the study identified the vulnerability to workers' rights abuse due to documentation status as a stressor. Individuals with no legal documentation are limited in the type of jobs they can secure, increasing stress and substance use risk. Lower socioeconomic status, less education, and documentation status reduce job prospects to ones that have a high risk of physical injury, which can lead to or exacerbate substance use that is prescribed and unprescribed. In the early 1900s, the Temperance Movement gained traction, leading to the prohibition of alcohol in the United States in 1920 (Moore & Gerstein, 1981). This had significant implications for permitted workplace substance

DOI: 10.4324/9781032708829-3

use, as many employers had to implement policies prohibiting the use of alcohol on the job. The Drug-Free Workplace Act of 1988 was an example of regulating substance use in the workplace through policy implementation. These policies, although intended for all illicit substances, were frequently cited for alcohol-related incidents, which contributed to the increased use of alternative substances.

As substance use became more widespread in the workplace, concerns about health and safety grew, and employers began to implement more stringent substance use policies. In the 1980s, the federal government passed legislation that required drug testing for certain industries, such as transportation and aviation (National Research Council, 1981). This trend continued into the 1990s and 2000s, with many companies implementing drug testing and zero-tolerance policies. As society has evolved and the risks associated with substance use during work have become better understood, policies have become more robust (ex: Omnibus Transportation Employee Testing Act of 1991). The significance of promoting a drug-free workplace cannot be understated as it pertains to health and safety, however, in some cases, these policies have had unintended consequences for minoritized employees (Oh et al., 2023). Examples of these consequences include disproportionate punish-ment for minoritized individuals compared to their White counterparts, increased frequency of drug testing, and early termination. These consequences also contribute to reduced access to treatment for minor-itized individuals (Oh et al., 2023).

Beyond the ways substance use shows up in the workplace, what is often not discussed is how the workplace influences substance use (Frone, 2006). Americans have adopted ideas of work life as "work hard, play hard" and "grind culture." These ways of looking at work have created an unhealthy and imbalanced work–life. Research has shown that work-stress contributes to excess alcohol use (Amaro, 2021; Frone, 2015, 2016) yet there is little research identifying what role workplace culture may play in alcohol consumption or substance use. Frone (2016) points out that there are very few studies that look at moderators and mediators for substance use and workplace stress. In addition, there is little research that takes a view of substance use from the perspective of workplace culture (Frone et al., 2022). Just like alcohol was used to assist with working conditions in the early 1900s, alcohol is now used to manage workplace stress. The difference is that use is now restricted to outside of work hours. Through the exploration of historical, social, and cultural factors, this chapter will highlight how substance use looks in the context of hiring inequity, workplace connecting, and work–life balance. It will take an inverse approach by reflecting how workplace culture influences substance use. Understanding how the workplace influences substance use from a cultural perspective promotes the development of innovative treatment plans from providers and highlights the need for more culturally responsive organizational intervention. There is a need for shifting workplace culture to be more inclusive and culturally responsive not only for people who may have substance use issues, but for society. It is my hope that this chapter will prompt more needed research on the area of culture as it pertains to workplace and substance use.

Hiring Inequity

In recent years, there has been growing recognition of the importance of cultural responsiveness in hiring practices. This involves considering the unique experiences and perspectives of diverse job candidates, including those who may have a history of substance use. Unfortunately, many employers continue to rely on outdated and incongruent hiring practices that can unfairly penalize individuals who use certain substances. The Drug-Free Workplace Act of 1988 requires federal organizations and non-federal organizations that receive federal funding conduct drug tests in their hiring practices. While drug testing can be an important tool for promoting workplace safety and productivity, it can also be a source of discrimination and bias. Businesses are becoming more aware of this as evidenced by the reduction in drug-testing. In October 2021, *TIME Magazine* published an article discussing the labor-shortage as a factor contributing to businesses ditching preemployment drug screening, high-lighting inequities for minoritized individuals as a key factor in the elimination of the practice. However, drug-testing remains a common practice for pre-employment. Employers using drug tests generally have a broad range of substances to test in their panel. Cannabis common as a tested substance but can remain in the body for several weeks after use depending on frequency and potency of use (Sharma et al., 2012). This can lead to situations where an individual is ruled out for a position based solely on a detected drug test for cannabis, even if they have not used the substance recently or are using it for medical purposes. Additionally, since cannabis is not yet fully regulated, products such as CBD may trigger a detected drug test. The cost and quality of drug tests is also a factor in hiring inequity when considering substance use. Continuing with the cannabis example, to obtain a more accurate understanding of when someone used the substance, a "THC Quantitative add-on" to the drug test will provide a percentage of THC that was detected in the sample. Though this may be helpful for companies to improve equity with their hiring practices, this add-on is an added cost to the business.

Consider the case of Daniel, a job candidate who uses medical cannabis to manage chronic pain. Daniel recently applied for a position at a local restaurant, and during the hiring process, was asked to submit to a drug test. Even though Daniel had not used cannabis for two weeks prior to the test, it came back detected, meaning there was cannabis in his system. As a result, the restaurant declined to offer Daniel the job.

Let's use the same example but with Sarah and change the substance. Sarah is a job candidate who uses cocaine recreationally on weekends. Sarah applied for the same position as Daniel at the local restaurant, and during the hiring process, was asked to submit to a drug test. Since cocaine is a substance that typically metabolizes quickly, Sarah's test came back undetected, meaning there were no illicit substances in her system at the time of the test, and she was offered the job. This situation highlights the incongruent nature of many drug testing policies, which do not consider the differences in metabolization times between different substances. It also demonstrates how outdated hiring practices can also unfairly penalize individuals who use certain substances.

In this case, Daniel is being unfairly penalized for his use of medically prescribed cannabis due to chronic pain while Sarah, who uses cocaine recreationally, is now employed. This example shows how hiring inequity can look based on substances due to how they metabolize in the body. It also emphasizes the limitations of drug testing as a required part of the hiring process. Some may think cocaine as an example is extreme, but alcohol can also be used in this example. Alcohol is metabolized in the body on average at a rate of 7 g/hr (Cederbaum, 2012). This means that it takes about 1 hour for the body to metabolize one "standard drink," which can be 12 ounces of beer, 5 ounces of wine, or 1.5 ounces of distilled spirits (80-proof). Additionally, there are several factors that contribute to alcohol metabolism such as body weight, physical health, age, and use of other medications. These factors can speed up or slow down the metabolism process; however, they are not considered when reviewing a drug test. Because of this, someone who has an active alcohol use disorder could provide an undetected drug test and be hired over someone who uses cannabis occasionally but has a detected drug test. Please note that the terms "detected" and "undetected" are being used intentionally as the terms "positive" and "negative" are considered value-laden terms and can contribute to continued maintenance of stigma in substance use.

It is also important to consider financial implications when using drug tests as a method for hiring practices. The more substances tested in a sample, the more expensive the costs of the tests are for the company. Even the method of sample collection (urine, hair, blood) can vary dramatically in price. Urine testing is the most common and least expensive method of drug testing, with an average cost of about $50 per test. Hair testing, on the other hand, is more expensive and can cost up to $150 per test. Blood testing is the most expensive method, with an average cost of about $200 per test. These price variations can translate to financial barriers in organizations, especially smaller ones with limited resources. Financial barriers such as this can contribute to organizations opting for less expensive testing methods which may be less accurate. For example, urine testing has a shorter detection window than hair testing, meaning it can only detect drug use in the past few days and sometimes less depending on the person's physiological characteristics. Because substances are constantly changing, there are instances where there is very little or no possibility for detection. Inhalants are an example of a substance often not considered and challenging to detect when using drug tests as a necessary component for job acquisition (Jain & Verma, 2016). Between financial barriers of companies and minimal accuracy of drug-tests, minoritized individuals are disproportionately removed from the pool of qualified candidates for jobs that use drug-testing as an entry point for a position. You might ask what this has to do with culturally responsive substance use treatment. As a provider, advocating for more equitable hiring practices is a systemic way to contribute to elevating the voices of individuals who have substance use backgrounds and struggle to find employment. As an organization, identifying more equitable screening processes for employees serves as a benefit to those who have a substance use history. As a system, understanding that these hiring practices are inequitable and contribute to covert and oppressive practices can contribute to the need for dismantling the status quo. As a researcher, studying correlations between substance use and hiring practices contributes data to the profession that helps move the needle in the direction of health equity. Drug testing is not a culturally responsive approach to determining employee qualifications. While it is a method that is beneficial for maintaining regulation in the workplace, it promotes discrimination and inequity among people who have a substance use history.

To address the issue of inequitable hiring practices related to substance use, there are several potential solutions. One approach is for employers to educate themselves on the limitations of drug testing methods as key determinants in hiring practices. This can include the differences in metabolization times between different substances and the different forms of drug tests. Another approach is for companies to simply consider these factors when interpreting drug test results for the purposes of hiring a possible candidate. This could involve leaders receiving training on the effects of different substances from substance use experts or working with industry groups to develop more nuanced drug testing policies. Additionally, companies and providers can advocate for alternative hiring practices that focus on skills and qualifications rather than drug use. For example, some employers have shifted away from drug testing altogether and instead rely on behavioral assessments, skills assessments, or other measures to evaluate job candidates. By adopting more culturally responsive and equitable hiring practices, employers can help to promote a more inclusive and diverse workplace while also improving equity among individuals who have been historically eliminated from selection due to these practices and further, limited in access to treatment as a result of these practices.

Inequitable hiring practices related to substance use can have far-reaching consequences for individuals and communities. By providing examples and data to illustrate the impact of these practices, we can raise awareness of the issue and work to promote more equitable and culturally responsive hiring practices. Through education, advocacy, and policy change, we can help to create a more just and inclusive environment for everyone.

Connection Over Cocktails

Corporate holiday parties, after-work cocktail hours, and extended off-site work events serve as avenues for fostering employee connections outside the confines of work. These gatherings aim to facilitate conversations among colleagues from different departments, encourage discussions unrelated to work, and alleviate work-related stress (Daniels et al., 2017). While these events are well-intentioned, they can inadvertently exclude individuals in recovery from substance use disorders due to the prevalence of alcohol and limited availability of non-alcohol-centered activities (Brown & Pehrson, 2019). It is also well documented that group dynamics play a large role in individual behavior (Park & Lee, 2011), which can lead to individuals engaging in substance use to be "accepted" into a group even if their personal behaviors are not in alignment with their group behaviors. Moreover, individuals who experience heightened anxiety in informal social settings may resort to excessive drinking as a means of coping with their anxious feelings (Anker & Kushner, 2019; Grant et al., 2005; Walukevich-Dienst et al., 2022).

Research has demonstrated a correlation between social anxiety and increased incidents of alcohol-related problems (Keough et al., 2016). Furthermore, individuals diagnosed with social anxiety disorder have a higher likelihood of developing alcohol use disorders, leading to diagnostic comorbidity (Grant et al., 2005; Johnson et al., 2000; Castillo-Carniglia et al., 2019). Seeing as we spend so much time in our work environments and with our coworkers, it can be inferred that individuals in work cultures that promote alcohol consumption may be more susceptible to over-consumption of substances to cope with their symptoms or developing an alcohol use disorder. Knowing this correlation as a provider can drastically improve treatment interventions that pertain to managing workplace culture and anxiety. This also can serve as rationale for an organizational culture shift to improve staff wellness by reducing alcohol related activities.

Additionally, it is important to note that alcohol, being a depressant, can exacerbate depressive symptoms. When individuals with depression consume alcohol in social settings, they are more susceptible to triggering depressive episodes (Keyes et al., 2019; Boden & Fergusson, 2011). To make the connection between addressing workplace culture and substance use, as of February 2023, it has been reported that approximately 32% of all adults ages 18–65 experience symptoms of anxiety and/or depression and that increases to almost half for people ages 18–24 (KFF analysis of U.S. Census Bureau, Household Pulse Survey, 2023). The correlation of increased depression and anxiety due to substance use should inform how workplace cultures involve alcohol in the attempt to connect colleagues (Caumiant et al., 2023). These events may very well be inadvertently increasing the mental health crisis. This highlights the need for awareness and sensitivity toward employees with mental health concerns in relation to alcohol consumption during workplace social events.

How might this relate to culturally responsive substance use treatment? Culturally responsive substance use treatment emphasizes the importance of tailoring treatment approaches to meet the unique needs and cultural backgrounds of individuals seeking help for substance use disorders. Understanding and addressing the impact of work culture norms, such as the prevalence of alcohol-centered social events, is crucial for providers working with individuals on their substance use journeys. This is especially important because we spend so much of our time in our work environments and with coworkers during and outside of work hours. Many people affectionately refer to coworkers as "work wife" or "work-husband" implying how much time they spend with their coworkers. Evolving from the perspective of limiting "self-care" to outside of work hinders one's ability to truly and comprehensively take good care of themselves given the significant overlap of workplace culture and personal life culture.

When working with someone in recovery, it is essential for providers to acknowledge and respect the client's triggers related to workplace social events. By helping individuals identify and develop strategies to reduce triggers associated with these events, providers can support their client's recovery process and promote sustained abstinence. Additionally, for individuals who experience anxiety in social settings, providers can assist in developing coping mechanisms that are alternatives to engaging in drinking behavior to manage anxiety specifically in those contexts. This individualized approach recognizes the unique challenges individuals may face and supports their overall well-being as it pertains to substance use. Viewing the whole person within the context of their different life environments contributes to the development of a culturally responsive substance use intervention. Consider the following as an example of how anxiety and substance use can show up in a corporate setting.

Derrick (He/Him), a newly hired staff, was excited to attend his company's annual holiday party. He has enjoyed getting to know his coworkers and was looking forward to engaging with them out of the office. Derrick saw the party as an opportunity to relax and enjoy a festive evening outside the confines of the office. Once Derrick arrived at the venue, he immediately heard laughter and music. When he walked into the space, he noticed a hosted bar with a wide variety of alcoholic beverages. Derrick, like many others, indulged in a few drinks to "loosen up" and celebrate the holiday season. However, as the evening progressed, Derrick found himself consuming alcohol more rapidly than intended, as many conversations were had near the bar area.

Unbeknownst to his colleagues, Derrick had been experiencing high levels of anxiety in this social setting. As a new employee, he wanted to make a good impression on his coworkers, but his desire to present "well" contributed to his increased alcohol consumption. As the effects of the alcohol intensified, his anxiety became more pronounced. He started feeling overwhelmed, uncomfortable, and struggled to engage in conversations. To quell his rising anxiety, Derrick continued to consume larger quantities of alcohol, hoping it would ease his symptoms.

Unfortunately, the combination of heightened anxiety and increased alcohol intake led to a regrettable incident. Derrick's judgment became impaired, and he unintentionally made inappropriate comments to a senior executive. The incident not only embarrassed Derrick, but it also strained his relationship with the executive and left Derrick feeling deeply remorseful. As a new hire he was intent on making a "good impression" but ended up embarrassing himself and dealing with immense amounts of guilt long after the holiday party.

This scenario underscores the importance of considering the potential consequences when planning corporate events that involve alcohol. Derrick's experience highlights the need for employers to be mindful of employees' diverse needs, including those who may struggle with anxiety or substance use concerns. Derrick did not have a substance use disorder or concerns with substance use in general. His anxiety symptoms influenced his overconsumption. By providing alternative activities and ensuring a welcoming and inclusive environment, companies can avoid inadvertently creating situations that may lead to alcohol-related incidents. In this context, it becomes essential for organizations to assess the impact of alcohol-centered events on their employees and consider alternative options. By offering a range of activities that cater to various interests and preferences, companies can foster an inclusive atmosphere where everyone feels comfortable and engaged. This approach not only helps prevent incidents like the one Derrick experienced but also promotes a positive work culture centered around respect and well-being.

It is important to note that it is not necessary to eliminate alcohol from corporate events, rather it is important to plan with alternatives in mind. An example of this could be having a fruit beverage station in addition to a hosted bar, or having a SodaStream area to increase excitement over alternative beverages without alienating employees who choose to abstain from alcohol. Additionally, activities at locations other than bars, such as tea houses or smoothie bars can provide space for people to make choices that are healthier for them and prevent potential alcohol-related incidents. Ultimately, Derrick's story serves as a reminder that planning corporate events that involve alcohol requires thoughtful consideration and sensitivity. By prioritizing the needs and potential vulnerabilities of employees, companies can create a work environment that is safe, inclusive, and supportive for all, ensuring that such events remain enjoyable and free from unintended consequences. These alternatives can also be suggested by providers to their clients as a culturally responsive intervention.

Incorporating alternative activities into social events can also showcase an organization's commitment to inclusivity and cultural responsiveness. Providing options beyond traditional happy hours or events in which alcohol is a prominently featured beverage demonstrates an understanding of the diverse needs and preferences of employees, including those in recovery or individuals who choose not to consume alcohol. Considering alternative options also benefits employees who may be pregnant. Consider this example as another potential situation related to alcohol as the beverage of choice at a corporate event.

Sophia (She/Her) was extremely excited about her company's Q3 closeout celebration. Every quarter, her company had an event to highlight employee "wins" and corporate successes. This was also an opportunity for Sophia to spend time outside of work with her colleagues and congratulate them on their accomplishments. She saw this as a great morale booster for the company and the reputation for the quarterly closeout celebration was that the company provided great food and great drinks. Since Sophia had been with the company for several years, she was familiar with the event and her colleagues knew her beverage of choice so well that someone always had a margarita waiting for her when she arrived. However, prior to the event, Sophia found out that she was pregnant. Sophia was still early in her pregnancy and had been talking with her therapist about her fear of miscarriage. As much as she wanted to fully embrace the festivities, she wasn't yet ready to share her pregnancy news with her coworkers. She wanted to wait until she was further along and had more time to prepare. Unfortunately, she knew the event would have alcohol, and since her colleagues knew that she enjoys a good margarita, it would be a challenge for her to participate without raising suspicions.

Sophia attempted to discuss options with her therapist. She didn't want to miss out on the Q3 closeout entirely, but she also didn't want to draw attention to her decision not to drink. On the day of the party, Sophia arrived with a well-thought-out strategy she discussed with her therapist. She arrived to the event early so that she would be able to place her order without people questioning her. Sophia also informed the bartender that she would not be drinking alcohol, and that if a coworker attempted to get her a drink, to make a non-alcohol margarita discreetly. This allowed her to have a drink in hand without raising any eyebrows. She mingled with her colleagues, engaging in conversations, and enjoying the festive event.

Throughout the evening, Sophia was careful not to draw attention to herself. She mingled strategically, avoiding discussions about alcohol or her drink choice. She focused on enjoying the company of her coworkers, celebrating their achievements, and sharing laughter. However, throughout the event, Sophia was constantly weary of being "exposed" or asked about her beverage. She enjoyed the event, but not nearly as much as she could have. She also left early, saying she had last minute deadlines she needed to get to, which still raised suspicion among her coworkers.

Sophia's experience, like Derrick's, also underscores the importance of considering the needs of all employees when planning corporate events involving alcohol. While her situation was unique, it highlights the significance of creating an inclusive environment where individuals can comfortably participate without feeling pressured to disclose personal information before they are ready. Her therapist planned with Sophia to help reduce suspicion around her avoidance of alcohol, but the anxiety Sophia experienced during the event was exacerbated. A culturally responsive intervention that targets the individual and the organization could be to discuss with Sophia her potential for involvement with planning this work event and offering suggestions of beverage stations or activities that promote inclusion for the company overall. This approach gives Sophia some control, autonomy, and potentially a meaningful impact on other colleagues who have concerns about consuming alcohol during the event. This approach also opens the opportunity for Sophia to increase her wellness through finding meaning in preventing other colleagues from feeling isolated like herself.

These examples are very different, but both reinforce the need for corporations to consider how they plan their events when the events have alcohol as a drink option and how providers can develop multilevel interventions that are culturally responsive. It is not enough to have mixers as the only beverage option alternative for employees who choose to abstain from alcohol. This consideration fosters an atmosphere of inclusivity and respect, ensuring that all employees can enjoy and engage in company events without feeling compelled to disclose sensitive information. Sophia's story serves as a reminder that employers should strive to create a work culture that respects employees' privacy and personal choices. By offering a variety of drink options and promoting an inclusive environment, companies can ensure that all employees, regardless of their circumstances, feel comfortable and included in corporate events.

Additionally, considering the values and expectations of the younger generation, such as Gen Z, in the corporate workforce is crucial (Kouloupoulos & Keldsen, 2014). Research indicates that Gen Z places a high value on social impact within work environments (Stillman & Stillman, 2017; Seemiller & Grace, 2017). By addressing the substance use crisis and providing alternative options that align with social causes, companies can demonstrate their commitment to making a positive impact and attract prospective employees who value inclusive practices and social responsibility.

In summary, incorporating cultural responsiveness into substance use treatment involves recognizing and addressing work culture norms, such as alcohol-centered social events. Providers can individualize their approach by assisting individuals in managing triggers and anxiety related to these events as well as offer innovative strategies that their clients can use to transform their work culture environment. From a corporate perspective, offering alternative activities demonstrates inclusivity and consideration for social causes, aligning with the values of younger generations. Workplace culture needs to be part of the conversation when discussing culturally responsive substance use treatment. These efforts contribute to a culturally responsive and supportive environment for individuals affected by mental health conditions and substance use disorders.

Work–Life Imbalance

As with many once in a lifetime worldwide events, the COVID-19 pandemic dramatically transformed the way we work forever, with many individuals transitioning to virtual hybrid working environments, and others working from home. While this shift has brought about numerous benefits, such as increased flexibility and reduced commuting time, the evolution of how we work due to COVID-19 has also introduced aspects of substance use that prior to the pandemic, were not part of the discussion or research. Though there is much push in society to have a good "work–life balance" it is clear there has not been success in attaining this balance with the ever-changing landscape of our world and the way we understand "work" post-pandemic. Furthermore, this work–life imbalance disproportionately affects marginalized individuals due to socioeconomic barriers that were intensified because of the pandemic. Lack of access to resources for childcare and disparities between office-based work and home-based work are a few examples (Pew Research Center, 2021). This worldwide pandemic has jolted society in ways that will be noted in history, both positively and negatively. Unfortunately, the work–life imbalance that has been worsened by COVID-19 has also increased substance use, which is reflected in the explosion of the addiction epidemic, which will be discussed further in chapter 4. This section focuses on the culmination of life responsibilities that have contributed to a significant imbalance of work and life, which has led to and continues to cause an increase in substance use.

The implementation of "virtual happy hours," where colleagues connect online to socialize and unwind, became a popular practice during the pandemic. While these events were intended to foster social connections lost during the pandemic and alleviate stress of the shared experiences from the pandemic, they inadvertently contributed to an increase in substance use. Consider the differences between an in-person happy hour versus a virtual happy hour. In-person happy hours have the benefit of leaving home and being in a "neutral environment," promoting the separation of work and home. Additionally, for people who do not generally drink, alcohol may not be present in the home, so a virtual happy hour promotes an individual going to purchase their own alcohol to participate, which leads to them having more alcohol in their home than under general circumstances. Additionally, at restaurants, there is someone making the beverage and managing the amount of alcohol that goes into the drink. This is not the case at home, causing individuals to potentially "overpour" their beverage. In some cases, companies have provided "mini-alcohol" packs as gifts for their employees to use for virtual happy-hours to foster connection. This also increases the access to alcohol in the home for individuals who may not drink often enough to have alcohol in the home.

This is not to say that having virtual happy hours is a "bad thing." It is important to note that individuals can regulate their drinking in their home, but often, the risks are not considered when suggesting a virtual happy hour. The desire for connecting overrides the consideration for people who may be experiencing higher levels of isolation due to the pandemic, which can lead to more excessive drinking behavior (Bickel, 2016). These higher levels of isolation are also more prevalent in minoritized and marginalized populations (Murthy, 2023). Moreover, the normalization of using substances as coping mechanisms in virtual happy hours can perpetuate a culture of substance use within work contexts as we have seen from the historical context regarding substance use and work at the beginning of this chapter.

Working from home has also blurred the boundaries between personal and professional life, often resulting in longer working hours and increased work demands. In the office setting, there are clear physical boundaries between work and personal life. Simple routines such as getting ready for work and driving to your workplace trigger your brain to shift focus. With this separation, it is easier to develop a work–life balance simply because there is a physical separation and more structure. Although getting out of bed and having a five-minute commute from your room to your home office may be rewarding for some, for others this shift can intensify stress levels and lead individuals to seek relief through substance use. The blurring of boundaries can cause individuals to feel an ongoing pressure to be available and productive outside of their general work hours, eroding their ability to relax and recharge. Consequently, this can lead to individuals resorting to substance use to detach from work-related stress and reclaim a sense of personal time (Tao et al., 2023; Tran et al., 2023). The initial detachment that came from traveling from home to work and back has dissipated, so finding another way to detach through substances increases. Studies have also shown a positive correlation between high work demands and substance use as a coping mechanism (Frone, 2015; Golden et al., 2006). As work becomes more all-encompassing of life, individuals may turn to substances to manage the pressure, creating a cycle of dependence and further exacerbating the work–life imbalance.

Conversely, the lack of social support and decreased accountability in a remote work environment can also contribute to increased substance use behaviors. For many people, having the flexibility of working from home allows for more productivity, more ownership of one's time, and the opportunity for individuals to improve their work–life balance through utilizing the flexibility of their work schedule to their advantage. For others, however, the lack of accountability and decreased social support opens the door for maladaptive coping strategies, increase in loneliness, and low motivation to engage in healthy pleasurable activities.

With schools and childcare facilities closing or operating at limited capacity during the pandemic, parents and guardians faced significant challenges in balancing work and caregiving responsibilities. People caring for multiple children had the burden of attempting to assist their children in virtual learning, with different teachers, on different virtual platforms, while managing their own work responsibilities. Parents lost their ability to have social support in childcare for children who were not yet school aged and had to manage to keep their toddlers entertained while running business meetings. Others, who did not have the ability to work remotely, had to take on the burden of taking time off, sometimes unpaid, to care for their children. In many cases, if parents or guardians did not take off work for childcare purposes, they had to take off work to care for their child who was exposed to another person with COVID while at school. These sacrifices led to job termination or loss of wages, making post-pandemic childcare impossible to afford and finding new employment to pay for childcare just shy of being laughable.

The childcare burden is an example of how virtual hybrid and work from home situations can be beneficial, but they do not mitigate the stress and overwhelm that parents and guardians experience from balancing work and childcare responsibilities. The Pew Research Center conducted a study in 2021 polling parents and guardians regarding their stress levels and childcare responsibilities. Data over-whelmingly showed that parents and guardians were more stressed, burned-out, and overwhelmed by the challenges of balancing work and childcare than pre-pandemic. Additionally, taking off work has con-tributed to significant financial burden in many marginalized households, threatening job, and home security for many families. These stressors and abrupt changes in life circumstances contribute to increased substance use behaviors. On top of the absence of reliable childcare options increasing parental stress, work performance is compromised. Working parents reported lack of productivity in the Pew Research Center study and noted that childcare responsibilities present unique challenges in work productivity. The lack of support systems and the increased strain on parents' time and energy further contributed to work–life imbalance and substance use.

The pandemic has overall disrupted our perception of time due to the elimination of daily routines. Even as the world shifts to a post-pandemic lifestyle, these disruptions continue to impact the way we navigate our lives. It has also opened doors for more opportunities and increased flexibility with the development of remote work. The loss of temporal structure, however, has led to challenges in managing workloads effectively and maintaining work–life boundaries. This ambiguity surrounding time can contribute to heightened stress levels and trigger substance use as a maladaptive coping mechanism. Recognizing and adapting to these changes in the concept of time are crucial in addressing work–life imbalance and its impact on substance use.

It may seem as though working remotely only has negative impacts as it pertains to substance use, however, the evolution of technology during the pandemic poses many opportunities to decrease health disparities and increase access to care through telemedicine. Because of this, retaining a balanced perspective is critical when considering these limitations and possible factors contributing to a work–life imbalance. As time progresses and we become more familiar with how to navigate the post-pandemic work landscape, mental health professionals can improve their treatment approaches to target the issues outlined in this section regarding working from home, substance use, and the general work–life imbalance. Aligning interventions with cultural awareness will increase the success of substance use treatment. One way to consider aligning interventions with cultural awareness would be to help the client by raising awareness of these mental loads that contribute to stress and are a direct result of the COVID-19 pandemic. The suggestion of "taking time off" to someone who is the primary income supporter of their family does not take into consideration their life circumstances or needs. Similarly, suggesting that someone engage in "self-care" is often a misstep culturally when considering the foundational barriers of blurring home and work. Instead, consider interventions that are concrete and practical to assist in setting work from home boundaries and promote a reduction in stress. Something as seemingly mundane as removing work email notifications from one's phone can serve as a stress reducing practice and simultaneously a boundary setting practice because it would then require the client to go to their desk for emails. Consider setting boundaries around times to be at their desk and times to walk away from their desk as additional micro-interventions to address some of the secondary contributing factors to their increased substance use.

The transition to virtual hybrid work and working from home due to COVID-19 has brought forth many aspects of work–life imbalance that contribute to increased substance use. By examining the influence of virtual happy hours, heightened work demands, blurring of work and home boundaries, childcare limitations, and changes in the concept of time, we can gain a deeper understanding of the challenges faced by individuals in developing and maintaining a healthy work–life balance. It is essential for treatment providers to acknowledge and address these issues by taking culture into consideration, ensuring that individuals receive comprehensive support in navigating work–life imbalance and its potential impact on substance use.

References

Amaro, H., Sanchez, M., Bautista, T., & Cox, R. (2021). Social vulnerabilities for substance use: Stressors, socially toxic environments, and discrimination and racism. *Neuropharmacology*, *188*, 108518. 10.1016/j.neuropharm.2021.108518

Anker, J. J., & Kushner, M. G. (2019). Co-occurring alcohol use disorder and anxiety: Bridging psychiatric, psychological, and neurobiological perspectives. *Alcohol Research: Current Reviews, 40*(1), arcr.v40.1.03. 10.35946/arcr.v40.1.03

Bickel, W. K., Moody, L., & Higgins, S. T. (2016). Some current dimensions of the behavioral economics of health-related behavior change. *Preventive Medicine, 92*, 16–23. 10.1016/j.ypmed.2016.06.002

Boden, J. M., & Fergusson, D. M. (2011). Alcohol and depression. *Addiction, 106*(5), 906–914.

Brown, R., & Pehrson, S. (2019). *Group processes: Dynamics within and between groups.* United Kingdom: Wiley.

Castillo-Carniglia, A., Keyes, K. M., Hasin, D. S., & Cerdá, M. (2019). Psychiatric comorbidities in alcohol use disorder. *The Lancet Psychiatry, 6*(12), 1068–1080. 10.1016/S2215-0366(19)30222-6

Caumiant, E. P., Fairbairn, C. E., Bresin, K., Rosen, I. G., Luczak, S. E., & Kang, D. (2023, March 9). Social anxiety and alcohol consumption: The role of social context. *Addictive Behaviors.* Advance online publication. 10.1016/j.addbeh.2023.107672

Cederbaum, A. I. (2012). Alcohol metabolism. *Clinics in Liver Disease, 16*(4), 667–685. 10.1016/j.cld.2012.08.002

Daniels, K., Watson, D., & Gedikli, C. (2017). Well-being and the social environment of work: A systematic review of intervention studies. *International Journal of Environmental Research and Public Health, 14*(8), 918. 10.3390/ijerph14080918

Frone, M. R. (2006). Prevalence and distribution of illicit drug use in the workforce and in the workplace: Findings and implications from a U.S. national survey. *Journal of Applied Psychology, 91*(4), 856–869. 10.1037/0021-9010.91.4.856

Frone, M. R. (2015). Relations of negative and positive work experiences to employee alcohol use: testing the intervening role of negative and positive work rumination. *Journal of Occupational Health Psychology, 20*(2), 148–160. https://doi.org/10.1037/a0038375

Frone, M. R. (2016). Work stress and alcohol use: Developing and testing a biphasic self-medication model. *Work and Stress, 30*(4), 374–394. 10.1080/02678373.2016.1252971

Frone, M. R., Casey Chosewood, L., Osborne, J. C., & Howard, J. J. (2022). Workplace supported recovery from substance use disorders: Defining the construct, developing a model, and proposing an agenda for future research. *Occupational Health Science, 6*(4), 475–511. 10.1007/s41542-022-00123-x

Furman, R., Ackerman, A. R., & Negi, N. J. (2012). Undocumented Latino immigrant men in the United States: Policy and practice considerations. *International Social Work, 55*(6), 816–822. 10.1177/0020872812450729.

Grant, B. F., Hasin, D. S., Blanco, C., Stinson, F. S., Chou, S. P., Goldstein, R. B., Dawson, D. A., Smith, S., Saha, T. D., & Huang, B. (2005). The epidemiology of social anxiety disorder in the United States: results from the national epidemiologic survey on alcohol and related conditions. *The Journal of Clinical Psychiatry, 66*(11), 1351–1361. 10.4088/jcp.v66n1102

Golden, T., Veiga, J., & Simsek, Z. (2006). Telecommuting's differential impact on work-family conflict: Is there no place like home? *Journal of Applied Psychology, 91*, 1340–1350. 10.1037/0021-9010.91.6.1340.

Jain, R., & Verma, A. (2016). Laboratory approach for diagnosis of toluene-based inhalant abuse in a clinical setting. *Journal of Pharmacy & Bioallied Sciences, 8*(1), 18–22. 10.4103/0975-7406.164293

Johnson, J. G., Cohen, P., Pine, D. S., Klein, D. F., Kasen, S., & Brook, J. S. (2000). Association between cigarette smoking and anxiety disorders during adolescence and early adulthood. *JAMA, 284*(18), 2348–2351. 10.1001/jama.284.18.2348

Kaiser Family Foundation (KFF). (2023). Latest federal data show that young people are more likely than older adults to be experiencing symptoms of anxiety or depression. *Kaiser Family Foundation.* https://www.kff.org/mental-health/press-release/latest-federal-data-show-that-young-people-are-more-likely-than-older-adults-to-be-experiencing-symptoms-of-anxiety-or-depression/

Keough, M. T., Battista, S. R., O'Connor, R. M., Sherry, S. B., & Stewart, S. H. (2016). Getting the party started—Alone: Solitary predrinking mediates the effect of social anxiety on alcohol-related problems. *Addictive Behaviors, 55*, 19–24.

Keyes, K. M., Allel, K., Staudinger, U. M., Ornstein, K. A., & Calvo, E. (2019). Alcohol consumption predicts incidence of depressive episodes across 10 years among older adults in 19 countries. *International Review of Neurobiology, 148*, 1–38.

Koulopoulos, T., & Keldsen, D. (2014). *The Gen Z effect: The six forces shaping the future of business*, 1st ed. Routledge. https://doi.org/10.4324/9781315230337

Murthy, V. H. (2023). *Our epidemic of loneliness and isolation: The U.S. surgeon general's advisory on the healing effects of social connection and community.* US Department of Health and Human Services.

National Research Council (US). (1981). Panel on alternative policies affecting the prevention of alcohol abuse and alcoholism. In M. H. Moore & D. R. Gerstein (Eds.), *Alcohol and public policy: Beyond the shadow of prohibition.* Washington, DC: National Academies Press (US). Temperance and Prohibition in America: A Historical Overview. Available from: https://www.ncbi.nlm.nih.gov/books/NBK216414/

Negi, N. J. (2011). Identifying psychosocial stressors of well-being and factors related to substance use among Latino day laborers. *Journal of Immigrant and Minority Health, 13*(4), 748–755. 10.1007/s10903-010-9413-x

Oh, S., Hodges, J., Salas-Wright, C., Smith, B., & Goings, T. C. (2023). Ethnoracial differences in workplace drug testing and policies on positive drug tests in the United States. *Drug and Alcohol Dependence, 247*, 109898. 10.1016/j.drugalcdep.2023.109898

Olson, S., & Gerstein, D. R. (1985). *Alcohol in America: Taking action to prevent abuse.* Washington, DC: National Academies Press (US). Available from: https://www.ncbi.nlm.nih.gov/books/NBK217463/

Park, H. S., & Lee, D. W. (2011). Alcohol-related social gatherings with coworkers: Intentions to behave and intentions to not behave. *Journal of Pacific Rim Psychology, 5*(2), 53–64. 10.1017/S1834490900000581

Pew Research Center. (2021, January 26). A rising share of working parents in the U.S. say it's been difficult to handle child care during the pandemic. *Pew Research Center*. https://www.pewresearch.org/short-reads/2021/01/26/a-rising-share-of-working-parents-in-the-u-s-say-its-been-difficult-to-handle-child-care-during-the-pandemic/

Seemiller, C., & Grace, M. (2017). Generation Z: Educating and engaging the next generation of students. *About Campus*, *22*(3), 21–26. 10.1002/abc.21293.

Sharma, P., Murthy, P., & Bharath, M. M. (2012). Chemistry, metabolism, and toxicology of cannabis: clinical implications. *Iranian Journal of Psychiatry*, *7*(4), 149–156.

Stillman, D. , & Stillman, J. (2017). *Gen Z @ work: How the next generation is transforming the workplace*, 1st ed. New York, NY: Harper Collins.

Tao, X., Liu, T., Giorgi, S., Fisher, C. B., & Curtis, B. (2023). Extended impact of the COVID-19 pandemic: Trajectories of mental health and substance use among U.S. adults, September 2020–August 2021. *Drug and Alcohol Dependence Reports*, *8*, 100186. 10.1016/j.dadr.2023.100186

Time. (n.d.). Workplace drug testing: What to know. *Time*. https://time.com/6103798/workplace-drug-testing/

Tran, D. D., Fitzke, R. E., Wang, J., Davis, J. P., & Pedersen, E. R. (2023). Substance Use, Financial Stress, Employment Disruptions, and Anxiety among Veterans during the COVID-19 Pandemic. *Psychological Reports*, *126*(4), 1684–1700. 10.1177/00332941221080413

Unde Ayvat, P., Aydın, O. N., & Oğurlu, M. (2012). Algoloji polikliniğine başvuran bel ağrılı hastaların risk faktörleri [Risk factors associated with lower back pain in the Polyclinic of Algology]. *Agri: Agri (Algoloji) Dernegi'nin Yayin Organidir = The Journal of the Turkish Society of Algology*, *24*(4), 165–170. 10.5505/agri.2012.38258

Walukevich-Dienst, K., Calhoun, B. H., Fairlie, A. M., Cadigan, J. M., Patrick, M. E., & Lee, C. M. (2022, Nov 28). Using substances to cope with social anxiety: associations with use and consequences in daily life. *Psychology of Addictive Behaviors*. PubMed PMID 36442020

Chapter 4

The "Now More Than Ever" Era of Addiction

COVID-19

A common phrase throughout the COVID-19 pandemic has been "now more than ever."

> "Now more than ever, we need to come together as a community."
> "In these uncertain times, now more than ever, we need to prioritize our health and well-being."
> "Now more than ever, it's important to stay informed about current events."
> "Now more than ever, we must take action to address climate change."
> "Now more than ever, we need to support small businesses and local economies."
> "Now more than ever, we must stand up against racism and discrimination."
> "In this age of digital connectivity, now more than ever, we need to safeguard our privacy."
> "Now more than ever, we must invest in education and technology to prepare for the future."
> "Now more than ever, we need to show empathy and kindness towards others."
> "In the midst of a global pandemic, now more than ever, we must practice good hygiene and social distancing." (pause, shouldn't we have always been practicing good hygiene?!)

To communicate a sense of urgency, the phrase "now more than ever" has been used so frequently for an array of different topics that it has lost its impact. Furthermore, its overuse has created a perspective that many of these issues are only *now* worth paying attention to when the truth is, we are well past the point of "now more than ever" and are currently in more of a "too little too late" stage. When making this statement in relation to substance use and substance use treatment, it suggests that substance use treatment is a new and urgent issue. Substance use treatment has been needed for decades, and it has been recognized as a public health

DOI: 10.4324/9781032708829-4

issue since at least the 1960s. The term "now more than ever" is already an oversaturated term, used almost as a scare tactic for people to "act now." Fear is intended as a trigger in our brain to act quickly in what we perceive to be dangerous situations, but using fear as an attempt to prompt action in a situation that is not immediately dangerous can dilute the fear response AND the action. Using fear is also antithetical to encouraging someone to engage in substance use treatment. Substance use disorders are a significant public health concern. According to the National Survey on Drug Use and Health, approximately 20 million Americans aged 12 and older had a substance use disorder in 2019. This number continues to increase, indicating that the need for substance use treatment was well established prior to the global pandemic. In fact, substance use is getting progressively worse and continues to disproportionately affect minoritized and racialized individuals. Despite the effectiveness of substance use treatment, access to treatment remains a challenge for many individuals. Barriers to treatment include stigma, lack of insurance coverage, and limited availability of treatment options in certain areas. Instead of simply stating that "now more than ever" we need to improve substance use treatment, practical and actionable steps need to be taken to adequately address these barriers.

Similarly, the term "now more than ever" as it pertains to the racial epidemic is absurd. Slavery. Jim Crow. Public lynchings. Hate crimes. These incidents were happening well before COVID-19, but if you were not directly impacted, you did not have to pay attention or know about them. With the world shutting down completely, leaving people with nothing to see but the news of horrible race-related murders, those who were previously not impacted were forced to see the reality of racism in real time. What's worse, the "now more than ever" era hasn't *actually* prompted significant behavior change in people due to its overuse. Hate crimes are still happening, Black and Brown people are still being killed by police, and racism is still very much alive and well. We, as a society, have been framing our issues as if everything is an emergency; but if everything is an emergency, then nothing is an emergency. Because of this, we need to make fundamental and systemic changes to try to undo the damage that has already been done.

It is unfortunate that the substance use treatment community is only recently coming to terms with the reality that racism plays a role in disproportionate substance use treatment in all capacities. From access to equitable substance use treatment, to substance use treatment outcomes, providers and treatment programs do not have culturally responsive interventions to meet the needs of the diverse substance use population. Some scholars believe that substance use "does not see race." Others posit that substance use treatment is equitable because the treatment is of the substance, not the person. Because of these invalidating and narrow perspectives, the issue of inequitable substance use treatment persists. Substance use disorders are often linked to underlying issues such as trauma, mental health disorders, and socioeconomic factors. Addressing these root causes is critical to preventing substance use disorders and ensuring long-term recovery. Overall, the phrase "now more than ever" mischaracterizes the need for substance use treatment. Substance use treatment has been needed for decades, and it remains a critical public health issue. By addressing the root causes of substance use disorders and ensuring access to culturally-informed evidence-based treatments, we can help individuals overcome substance use disorders and improve public health outcomes. In order to address these root causes, understanding the intersectionality of the COVID-19 pandemic and the racial epidemic will provide a truly comprehensive understanding of the addiction epidemic. Additionally, it will make clear how addressing these root causes can open the door for equitable and culturally responsive substance use treatment for other marginalized individuals.

The COVID-19 Pandemic

In August 2019, I was informed that I had been nominated to serve on the American Psychological Association's (APA) Membership Board. The term was for 3 years, and it would require attendance at several meetings located in Washington, DC. I was notified that I had been elected to the APA Membership Board in December 2019 and my term would start in January 2020. The first meeting to be held in DC was scheduled for March 20, 2020. This consolidated meeting was intended to provide all people serving on boards and committees of APA with an opportunity to connect, plan, and coordinate their initiatives for the year. Additionally, there would be opportunities to collaborate across boards and committees to help move forward shared initiatives. This was my first time serving in APA governance as a professional, and I was excited about the prospect of engaging in thought leadership across the organization. I scheduled my flight and hotel in January 2020, and planned to meet with several colleagues while in DC. Two weeks before the consolidated meeting, consolidated meeting participants were notified via email of the raising concern about coronavirus. As of March 6, 2020, the email indicated "no confirmed cases in Washington, DC" and "during the meeting, we will ask attendees to fist-bump or elbow bump or use other non-contact and culturally-sensitive greetings rather than hugs and handshakes." The plan was to press on with the meeting but proceed with caution. I remember a dear friend and colleague sharing that she was in DC for an APA leadership event on March 9, 2020, just 10 days before I would arrive in DC for the consolidated meeting.

On March 11, 2020, I received an email stating that "based on the evolving circumstances surrounding the COVID-19 outbreak and a commitment to public health, the American Psychological Association has decided to cancel the in-person Consolidated Meeting." Furthermore, the email indicated that ALL APA in-person meetings would be canceled through April 30, 2020. March 11, 2020, will be a day marked with one of the largest worldwide pandemics in history. I clearly remember the raising concern within myself and among my colleagues, family, and friends, when the world shut down.

The COVID-19 pandemic, caused by the novel coronavirus SARS-CoV-2, began in late 2019 and has since had a profound impact on the world. The first cases of COVID-19, categorized as a "pneumonia-like" illness were reported in Wuhan, Hubei Province, China, in December 2019. After further investigation, the illness was identified as a novel coronavirus, and formally named SARS-CoV-2. In January 2020, The World Health Organization (WHO) was informed about the outbreak in Wuhan and began monitoring the situation closely. At this point, the virus had begun to spread within China and to other countries. On January 30, 2020, the WHO declared the COVID-19 outbreak a Public Health Emergency of International Concern (PHEIC). This was the first formal acknowledgment of the global threat posed by the virus. On March 11, 2020, the WHO declared COVID-19 a worldwide pandemic, signifying the global spread and severity of the disease. Governments across the globe began to implement various measures to contain the virus. Mandated lockdowns occurred, forcing schools and employers to shut down their establishments and encouraging people to stay in their homes. Mandated travel restrictions were put in place, as an attempt to ensure people did not spread the virus if they were contagious and reduce the rapidly spreading illness. Social distancing guidelines were established, which meant people were required to keep no less than 6 feet of distance between one another if gathering, masks were to be worn when in public, and people were strongly encouraged to refrain from any physical contact with other people.

Unfortunately, this was not enough to keep COVID-19 from spreading. Between March and April 2020, the number of COVID-19 cases and deaths rose rapidly worldwide, particularly in Europe and the United States. Healthcare systems began to face significant strain with an influx of patents with COVID-19 needing care. Many countries did not have the infrastructure necessary to provide treatment to individuals who were sick, and many healthcare systems weren't completely sure what to do to help patients coming in for treatment. Ironically, even with the influx of patients in hospitals and the rising death toll, between May and June 2020, several countries began easing lockdown restrictions and implementing phased reopening plans. The economy had been severely damaged as a result of the preceding lockdowns and restrictions, so countries used these reopening plans and ease of restrictions in hopes of revitalizing their economies while also maintaining precautionary measures. Regrettably, because of these attempts to phase out the lockdowns, outbreaks continued to occur in different parts of the world. Some countries began to experience a "second wave" of infections, triggering the reintroduction of restrictions and local lockdowns.

By November 2020, multiple pharmaceutical companies announced their development of COVID-19 vaccines. The regulatory approval process began and was expedited to attempt to stop the spread of COVID-19. Upon the new year, in January 2021, the global vaccination effort and campaigns to promote getting vaccinated gained momentum, but challenges related to vaccine supply, distribution, and vaccine hesitancy began to emerge. It should be noted that the United States has a long history of vaccine deception and the use of unethical practices in minoritized and racialized populations. Between the years 1932 and 1972, the U.S. Public Health Service conducted what is infamously named the "Tuskegee Syphilis Study" or "experiment." In this experiment, Black men who were diagnosed with syphilis were denied available medical treatment for syphilis, and instead were used as test subjects to study the progression of the disease in the human body. They were intentionally misinformed about the study and availability of curing medication, and many died as a result of not receiving available treatment. Another example is Henrietta Lacks. In 1951, the cells of Henrietta Lacks, a Black woman, were taken and studied in medical research without her consent. She was diagnosed with cervical cancer and during one of her biopsies, some of her cells were taken and grown separately in a lab without her consent. She passed in 1951 of cervical cancer, and her cells continued to be studied without the consent of her family. The use of her cells were instrumental in the development of the polio vaccine and cancer research advancements, but there was no credit given to her or her family for her contributions to science. It is because of these, and many other government-led studies that targeted Black and Brown individuals, that the intersection of COVID-19, the racial epidemic, and the addiction epidemic all play a role in understanding how to attain and deliver culturally responsive substance use treatment.

By the time vaccines were being distributed, new variants of the virus, such as the Alpha, Beta, Gamma, and Delta variants, were identified, which lead to concerns about their increased transmissibility and potential impact on vaccine efficacy. Between March and May 2021, vaccination programs continued to expand, and more countries administered vaccines to individuals who had a desire to obtain the vaccination. Some countries experienced declining case numbers, leading again to the easing of restrictions, while others continued to experience surges in infections. By June 2021, many countries had more success with getting people vaccinated, which resulted in decreased hospitalizations and deaths in vaccinated individuals. However, vaccination rates continued to vary worldwide due to the barriers to access, limited supply, and vaccination apprehension, and some regions continued to face challenges in controlling the virus. The health disparities among marginalized individuals have also become more salient because of the barriers listed above, and there is a disproportionate number of Black and Brown individuals who continue to die from the virus. Despite the expectation of many individuals that COVID-19 will "eventually be akin to the flu," the disparities that have been worsened because of COVID-19 remain. The marginalized populations who have yet to receive access to the vaccine are still struggling. The social determinants of health that have been further exposed to the public are still an issue. Minoritized communities are still in some ways battling the pandemic as if it is 2020.

Efforts to vaccinate the global population continue with a focus on increasing vaccine accessibility, distribution, and coverage in less developed regions. Additionally, ongoing research and surveillance by the WHO continue to help monitor the effectiveness of vaccines against new variants and guide public health strategies. The years 2020 through 2023 have shown us that the situation regarding the COVID-19 pandemic can evolve rapidly. It has also made abundantly clear the overwhelming disparities that minoritized populations experience. Large amounts of federal grant funding have been released to promote health equity and reduce health disparities among minoritized and marginalized groups, but realistically, for change to occur, systems and institutionalized racism need to be addressed, targeted, and dismantled. Culturally responsive substance use treatment involves addressing these much needed structural and systemic issues as well.

The Racial Epidemic

The 1920s had key cultural impacts including prohibition, which has had a huge impact on how society views and treats alcohol, women's rights, and social justice to name a few. As such, it makes sense that a century later, 2020 was a year intent on leaving a lasting impression. As mentioned, COVID-19 forced the world to stop. It forced the world to stop and pay attention to what was happening in our homes, our lives, our communities, and all around us. COVID-19 kept us from being able to ignore tragedies by busying ourselves with work. It kept us from inadvertently ignoring homelessness and global warming. COVID-19 made clear aspects of our lives and society that we were comfortable "not knowing." This is again why the "now more than ever" phrase is a mischaracterization of what is and has been happening around us for centuries.

Amid another COVID-19 surge, at the height of confusion and stay-at-home orders, many of us witnessed inhumanity in relatively real time. On May 25, 2020, a Black man in Minneapolis, Minnesota, was approached by police after they received a call that he bought cigarettes with a counterfeit $20 bill. Within 18 minutes of the call, the man, George Floyd, was murdered. We, as a society, watched the video of police officer Derek Chauvin pressing his knee on George Floyd's neck. We, as a society, watched as George Floyd gasped for air to call for his mother and say, "I can't breathe." We, as a society, watched as George Floyd lay unconscious under the police officer's knee, lifeless. This was, effectively, a public lynching. Many would say that this horrific murder displayed on television is what prompted the racial epidemic. Protests and outrage from all over were broadcast. #BlackLivesMatter was one of the most used hashtags in 2020. "Now more than ever" flooded media outlets calling for racial equity. Everyone saw this senseless act, and people were outraged. Concerningly, this was not the first time a Black person was senselessly murdered. This was not the first time Black lives *didn't* matter. On February 26, 2012, 8 years prior to George Floyd's murder, a 17-year-old Black child named Trayvon Martin was murdered by a neighbor. News outlets followed the story, but the audience was not held captive by a worldwide pandemic. Some might argue that Trayvon's story is different as he was killed by a neighbor, not a police officer. Others might say that though George Floyd's murder was horrific, it has nothing to do with culturally responsive substance use treatment. That perception is an example of a structural problem and reflects a lack of awareness about how institutionalized racism and systemic oppression work.

There are several instances of Black and Brown individuals being wrongfully murdered by police, so many so that it is disproportionate enough to cause a national alternative number to 911 during a mental health crisis, 988. When I saw the George Floyd video, I sobbed. As a Black person, to see the lack of care for Black life, to feel the pain so personally, and to feel hopeless because of the color of my skin, gives me a deep and personal understanding of why marginalized individuals engage in substance use. I was committed to contribute my expertise in a way that reduced disparities and dismantled racism at a system level however I could. Around this time of George Floyd's death, I came across a local story about Miles Hall. Miles Hall was a young Black man who was well known in his community and his family was well established in their neighborhood. Miles grew up in the same area and had good relationships with neighbors and people in the community. He was a high school graduate and aspiring musician. Although Miles had a mental health condition, his family made all attempts to obtain support from mental health agencies, hospitals, and the local community. Miles's family felt safe in their neighborhood and with the police, so when they called the police during one of Miles's mental health crises, they expected the police to assist Miles as they had in the past to obtain care for his mental health condition. Unfortunately, and devastatingly, the police arrived in Miles's neighborhood after this phone call and killed him. Miles Hall, a 19-year-old young Black man, was killed by police during a mental health crisis on June 2, 2019. Miles was killed almost exactly 1 year before George Floyd, but admittedly I had no idea. This was a situation in my community, and I had no idea until I was captive just like everyone else from COVID-19.

I share Miles's story for a variety of reasons. It is important to know that Black people are disproportionately killed due to systemic and institutionalized racism. Several studies showcase the false perception that Black people are more dangerous (Trawalter et al., 2008; Wilson et al., 2017), the tendency for people to treat Black children as adults (Cooke & Halberstadt, 2021; Goff et al., 2014), and the idea that Black people can tolerate higher levels of pain than others (Hoffman et al., 2016). Additionally, the mistrust of doctors and medical professionals in minoritized communities because of unethical medical practices and lack of adequate medical treatment contributed to those same people within those minoritized communities developing preexisting conditions that then made them more vulnerable to COVID-19. It is also important to note that regardless of how "good" a Black person is, they are still subject to institutionalized racism, which can lead to their death. Miles's story is an example of that along with many other stories like his. I share Miles's story also because these stories often get missed due to systemic racism. Since learning of his story, I have participated in raising awareness and utilized my own platform to contribute to dismantling racism in mental health and substance use treatment by elevating the concept of cultural responsiveness in mental health and substance use treatment practices. It is not enough to name institutionalized racism, there must be a willingness for society to accept this truth, and part of the acceptance is learning of the untold, unseen, and unheard stories. Miles's story birthed the Miles Hall Lifeline Act in California, which is associated with the 988-crisis line. This line is now national and has been introduced into legislation under varying names, but in California, it is named after a young Black man who was killed by police during a mental health crisis. His story was a contributing factor in the need for an alternative to 911.

The intersectionality of COVID-19 and the racial epidemic is unique. It is because of COVID-19 that there is an acknowledgement of the racial epidemic, a push for dismantling institutional racism, and an emphasis on Diversity, Equity, and Inclusion (DE&I). COVID-19 has also placed an established concept, Social Determinants of Health (SDoH), into a more central focus as a component of improving health equity. SDoH provide a systemic framework for how institutional racism and oppression play a role in health outcomes of marginalized and minoritized individuals. The Office of Disease Prevention and Health Promotion defines Social Determinants of Health as "conditions in the environments where people are born, live, learn, work, play, worship, and age that affect a wide range of health, functioning, and quality-of-life outcomes and risks (Healthy People 2030 US department of Health and Human services)." Some examples of SDoH include racism, discrimination, education, income, job opportunities, language and literacy skills, housing, safety, and polluted air and water. All of which have been made clear as issues due to the pandemic. Take this example of how SDoH disproportionately impacts minoritized individuals and contributes to the increased risk of substance use.

Isabella (She/Her) is a first-generation Latinx American, and her primary language spoken at home and the first language she learned is Spanish. The community in which she lives is also primarily Spanish-speaking. She learned most of her English from primary school, but due to the limited English many of the students spoke, her school regularly underperformed in academics. When Isabella got to high school, she struggled significantly with her academics. Because her parents did not speak English, they were limited in the work they could obtain. As a result, Isabella began working to help with finances at home, and often did not have time to complete homework assignments or engage in after-school activities.

When Isabella graduated from high school, her mother became ill, but it was unclear what her mother was ill from. No one in Isabella's family had medical knowledge, and their medical co-pay was extremely high, keeping Isabella's mother from seeking medical treatment. Additionally, as a Catholic family, Isabella's parents prioritized praying over her mother's illness. Isabella's mother often complained that the few times she did visit a medical professional, they would tell her to limit her gluten intake and take medications but would never listen to her or they often misunderstood what she was saying bothered her. Between Isabella's job, attempts to serve as her mother's translator, and her mother's illness, Isabella began developing migraines. She often had to "power through" the migraines to keep from missing work, but she struggled to balance everything in her life.

Eventually, Isabella went to a medical professional and shared her difficulty concentrating, irritability, and frequent migraines. She was prescribed medications but was not scheduled for any follow-up. Unfortunately, Isabella was experiencing symptoms of depression, but because she did not have the words to adequately describe her symptoms, she was quickly dismissed by the medical professional. A friend of Isabella's suggested she consider cannabis to help with her migraines. She began vaping and found that her depressive symptoms were lifting, but she experienced other symptoms such as forgetfulness and apathy. Since she could not afford the medication prescribed to her, nor could she afford to attend a follow-up appointment, she continued to vape cannabis.

This example highlights several social determinants of health that contribute to health disparities and substance use among minoritized and marginalized individuals in several different ways. Cultural and language barriers contribute to limited access to healthcare and health information. They also can lead to miscommunication and misunderstandings between patients and providers. The healthcare system is challenging for even the most educated and well-resourced individuals, so adding language barriers creates a higher level of complexity and onus on the part of the client. Additionally, lack of cultural responsiveness and awareness to provide culturally appropriate interventions and develop a culturally appropriate conceptualization of Isabella's symptoms and her mother's illness can lead to misdiagnosis and improper medical treatment. This leads to mistrust of the medical system and lack of appropriate and adequate healthcare. Moreover, Isabella's socioeconomic status prevents her family from having equitable housing and healthcare, and requires Isabella to get her own job early, preventing her from obtaining post-secondary education.

As illustrated in Isabella's example, social determinants of health play a crucial role in influencing an individual's health outcomes, including access to and outcomes of substance use treatment. When examining substance use treatment in marginalized communities, several SDoH play a significant role in the substance use treatment disparities (Yale Medicine, 2021). Individuals belonging to marginalized communities often experience higher poverty rates, limited educational opportunities, and reduced access to quality healthcare (Baah et al., 2019). These socioeconomic factors can create barriers to accessing substance use treatment, such as lack of insurance coverage, transportation challenges, or financial constraints. Discrimination and stigma also contribute to disproportionate and inequitable substance use treatment among marginalized communities. Although research shows that overall, people who report substance use are often treated inequitably, minoritized individuals are often dealing with the stigma of substance use in addition to the systemic racism in the medical industry (Colistra et al., 2023; Feagin & Bennefield, 2014). These negative attitudes experienced by marginalized individuals from medical providers lead to limited access to treatment services, fear of seeking help, and reduced quality of care.

Substance use disorders are also often linked to unstable housing situations and homelessness. Because marginalized communities already face higher rates of housing insecurity, obtaining access to consistent and appropriate substance use treatment presents an additional barrier (Camara et al., 2022). As mentioned, the layered nature of SDoH and substance use is a clear contributing factor to the increased likelihood of substance use due to homelessness. Increased vulnerability and limited resources for marginalized groups then folds into lack of adequate culturally responsive substance use treatment. In Chapter 9, I will go into more detail regarding this additional barrier that marginalized communities carry a burden of historical trauma resulting from systemic oppression, colonization, or intergenerational trauma. These experiences also contribute to higher rates of substance use disorders and pose unique challenges in substance use treatment, requiring culturally sensitive and trauma-informed approaches.

The racial epidemic and substance use in the "now more than ever" era has also shed more light on how the criminal justice system has continued to play a prominent role in systemic racism and disproportionate substance use treatment. Addiction has been criminalized for decades and has actively targeted communities of color. One of the most notable depictions of this is the "war on drugs" from the 1970s and subsequently, the "crack epidemic" in the 1980s. The criminalization of addiction, fueled by the "war on drugs," contributed to the era of mass incarceration, disproportionately affecting communities of color (Tomlin & Völlm, 2022; Wells & Kavanaugh, 2022). Because marginalized communities often face higher rates of criminal justice system involvement, instead of receiving culturally responsive substance use treatment, they receive punitive treatment that also does not address the external factors such as systemic oppression that contribute to disproportionate rates of incarceration despite reports of substance use comparable to their White counterparts.

Alexandra's Law, a bill that was introduced to California's senate in 2023 (California State Senate, n.d.), is another example of how systemic racism continues to quell opportunities for culturally responsive substance use treatment, and instead, turns to the criminal justice system as a solution for substance use disorders. The proposed bill would require individuals who are convicted of a fentanyl-related offense to be notified that if someone dies as a "direct consequence" of their fentanyl-related offense, that the convicted individual could be charged with homicide.

Once again, we see criminalization over treatment without consideration for how to provide care to the person with the substance use disorder. In addition to the criminalization over treatment and prevention, a law like this does not apply to medical providers prescribing deadly amounts of fentanyl. It also does not address the several extenuating circumstances of the person who engaged in the substance use. The person using substances may have ingested other substances in addition to the substance sold to them, they may have an underlying medical condition, it may have been a suicide attempt, among other things. The concern is that this law does not address any issue, all it does is place a homicide conviction on someone who also likely needs treatment. It does not bring the deceased back to life, and it does not stop the substances from circulating the street (remember, these are prescribed medications). Criminalizing any form of substance use behavior historically has contributed to a disproportionate amount of minoritized individuals being incarcerated. It also has yet to show any benefit for reduction in substance use disorders. Addressing these social determinants of health is crucial in improving substance use treatment outcomes in marginalized communities.

Because these issues are so multidimensional, if we are going to continue to use the "now more than ever" phrase, now more than ever, we need to address them from a multidimensional approach. Increasing access to affordable healthcare services, including substance use treatment, through policy changes and expanding insurance coverage is a start to addressing the needs of minoritized individuals experiencing healthcare deficiencies. Reducing stigma and discrimination through education, raising awareness, and promoting inclusive and culturally competent care through practical interventions can increase the likelihood that these underserved individuals will seek treatment. Implementing housing programs and supportive services to address housing instability and homelessness among individuals with substance use disorders will provide basic needs to individuals and allow them to focus on obtaining consistent and culturally responsive substance use treatment. Incorporating trauma-informed approaches and culturally sensitive interventions to address historical trauma and improve engagement and retention in substance use treatment among minoritized individuals is also necessary because as mentioned, if the historical and systemic issues are not acknowledged, they cannot be addressed. Furthermore, promoting diversion programs and alternatives to incarceration for individuals with substance use disorders would reduce the negative consequences of criminal justice involvement. Dismantling the institutionalized racist practices look like contributing to the interventions listed above. By recognizing and addressing these social determinants of health at a system level, substance use treatment can become more equitable, accessible, and effective for individuals belonging to marginalized communities, ultimately improving health outcomes, and reducing health disparities overall.

The Addiction Epidemic

The "now more than ever" era has exposed several long-standing issues society has had but has not necessarily addressed. COVID-19 in and of itself was a whirlwind for society, and amid the worldwide pandemic, several epidemics rose to the top of consciousness. The racial epidemic presented us with a need for massive social change, and the social determinants of health framework is a way in which society is attempting to take a more comprehensive approach to dismantling systemic racism. This will be discussed more in Chapter 6. The addiction epidemic has also provided a push for society to bring to light what has been done in darkness for decades. As mentioned, COVID-19 caused us to take a front row seat at the show as it pertains to how addiction has crippled our society. The addiction epidemic and the COVID-19 pandemic have truly eroded the layers covering a pre-existing crisis. Addiction, long prevalent and overlooked, has been exacerbated by the global health crisis, and has resulted in a confluence of challenges that can no longer be ignored.

As with the racial epidemic, COVID-19 has had a transformative effect on the addiction landscape. Socioeconomic disparities, trauma, mental health challenges, and limited access to treatment have been constant barriers to adequate substance use treatment. However, isolation, economic upheaval, and disrupted support systems resulting from the pandemic have compounded the vulnerability and desperation experienced by individuals who have substance use disorders. These additional factors have also contributed to the increase in individuals who cope using substances and those who have developed substance use disorders over the course of the pandemic.

Research shows that isolation contributes to adverse mental health outcomes (Cosco et al., 2021; Sobalvarro et al., 2023). Neglect is considered a contributing factor for increased risk of violence victimization and perpetration for youth in the well-known Adverse Childhood Experiences (ACE's) study (Centers for Disease Control and Prevention, 2021). Neglect has also been associated with increased risk of youth alcohol use and misuse and further leading to alcohol dependence (Zhen-Duan et al., 2023). One of the most impactful outcomes of COVID-19 was isolation. Although it was for the safety of ourselves and those around us, COVID-19 is marked with one of the most profound displays of isolation we have seen in our lifetime. The isolation experienced from COVID-19 is one factor that has truly expanded the addiction epidemic as evidenced by the continuous research being published regarding the increase in substance use behavior and drug overdose since the beginning of the pandemic (Chacon et al., 2021). Many individuals have noted their onset of substance use or increase in substance use is a way to cope with COVID-19 according to the Centers for Disease Control and Prevention.

The isolation people have experienced because of COVID-19 has also negatively impacted social support. When the world shut down, community meetings for individuals in recovery were no longer accessible. Though community support meetings pivoted and quickly developed an online presence and access like many employers, the initial impact of abruptly losing a social network and having no alternatives served as a unique barrier that only occurred due to a worldwide health crisis. Individuals who did not previously engage in substance use behavior reported starting in an attempt to cope, so imagine what it was like for individuals hanging on by a thread to their recovery. Imagine what it was like for individuals confident in their recovery because they had a solid support system. The pandemic snatched recovery from those who had it and contributed to addiction for those who did not. The addiction epidemic expanded beyond people who have substance use disorders and crippled the already lacking substance use treatment that was available. If any situation warrants the use of "now more than ever," the elimination of social support would be it.

The COVID-19 pandemic also placed significant strain on healthcare systems. Hospitals were quickly overcrowded from positive COVID-19 cases and medical complications because of COVID-19 in addition to the medical conditions that people experienced outside of COVID-19. The healthcare strain due to the pandemic extended to addiction treatment services. The lockdown mandates and the social distancing mandates reduced addiction treatment facility capacity by forcing facilities to maintain empty rooms for social distancing purposes, and prevented staff from providing in-person sessions if the facility was not initially deemed an "essential service." Prior to the pandemic, obtaining addiction treatment services was limited. With the additional restrictions and new limitations, access to treatment for addiction services was almost non-existent, leaving people with little to no support for substance use treatment.

The pandemic also led to widespread job losses due to business closures. Many businesses not deemed as an "essential service" had to shut their doors completely, leaving no opportunity to gain revenue. The economic instability of the world due to the closure of non-essential businesses such as restaurants, hotels, and corporate offices left many people without jobs or income. The Consumer Financial Protection Bureau (2022) conducted its Making Ends Meet 2022 survey and found that although it is recommended to maintain 6 months of savings for living expenses to have in case of financial emergencies, only approximately 27% of Americans reported having that much saved. Many individuals experienced financial strain, unemployment, and a loss of income. Financial stress is a known risk factor for substance abuse and addiction (Cho et al., 2023). Drinking to cope with the financial stress of job loss or financial strain exacerbated the already mounting addiction epidemic, making it even more challenging to address or attempt to control through treatment.

Increased access to substances is one factor of the pandemic that worsened the addiction epidemic that may have been overlooked. Grocery delivery systems skyrocketed during the pandemic to maintain profitability and get household essentials to consumers without having to take on risk of contracting COVID-19. This economic shift opened the door for alcohol delivery through grocery stores, restaurants, and liquor stores. Additionally, in areas where cannabis is legal, cannabis delivery systems became more prevalent. The stigma of engaging in excessive substance use and the stigma of what types of substances were being used were removed due to delivery systems. You now can smoke in your own home and drink as much as you feel without the social stigma or judgement because no one is watching. Pairing isolation-disrupted social support, and increased ease of access of substances made the growth of the addiction epidemic almost inevitable.

The phrase "now more than ever" used to illicit a sense of urgency and action in society, but it's due to its overuse has been rendered impotent. The COVID-19 pandemic, the racial epidemic, the addiction epidemic, and the intersectionality of them all need to be key points of consideration when engaging in culturally responsive substance use treatment. Noting that none of these epidemics came about because of COVID-19, but instead were made more visible to an international audience, provides acknowledgment to those who have been impacted by these epidemics long before COVID-19. It should not have to take a worldwide pandemic for society to pay attention to injustice in the world. Nor should it take a worldwide pandemic to reflect the harsh realities of, and challenges with, people who have substance use disorders. Unfortunately, though, that is exactly what happened. Instead of using COVID-19 as a *reason* to act in any of these areas, it is critical to acknowledge the history of the racial epidemic and addiction epidemic. Acknowledgement is the first step in addressing the issues and truly moving toward meaningful and sustainable systemic change. "Now more than ever" is a thing of the past. We are well beyond "now more than ever," the next step is actually putting words into action.

References

Baah, F. O., Teitelman, A. M., & Riegel, B. (2019). Marginalization: Conceptualizing patient vulnerabilities in the framework of social determinants of health-An integrative review. *Nursing Inquiry*, *26*(1), e12268. 10.1111/nin.12268

California State Senate. (n.d.). Senate Bill No. 44. California State Senate. https://sd34.senate.ca.gov/sb-44

Camara, C., Surkan, P. J., Van Der Waerden, J., Tortelli, A., Downes, N., Vuillermoz, C., & Melchior, M. (2022). COVID-19-related mental health difficulties among marginalized populations: A literature review. *Global Mental Health (Cambridge, England)*, *10*, e2. 10.1017/gmh.2022.56

Centers for Disease Control and Prevention. (2021). Adverse childhood experiences (ACEs). *CDC - Violence Prevention*. https://www.cdc.gov/violenceprevention/aces/index.html

Chacon, N. C., Walia, N., Allen, A., Sciancalepore, A., Tiong, J., Quick, R., Mada, S., Diaz, M. A., & Rodriguez, I. (2021). Substance use during COVID-19 pandemic: Impact on the underserved communities. *Discoveries (Craiova, Romania)*, *9*(4), e141. 10.15190/d.2021.20

Cho, J., Sussman, S., Kechter, A., Vogel, E. A., Barrington-Trimis, J. L., Unger, J. B., & Leventhal, A. M. (2023). Alcohol use and life stressors during the COVID-19 pandemic: A longitudinal study of young adults. *Journal of Substance Use*, Advance online publication. 10.1080/14659891.2023.2183909

Colistra, A. L., Ward, A., & Smith, E. (2023). Health disparities, substance-use disorders, and primary-care. *Primary Care*, *50*(1), 57–69. 10.1016/j.pop.2022.11.001

Consumer Financial Protection Bureau. (2022). Insights from making ends meet survey 2022. *Consumer Financial Protection Bureau*. https://www.consumerfinance.gov/data-research/research-reports/insights-from-making-ends-meet-survey-2022/

Cooke, A. N., & Halberstadt, A. G. (2021). Adultification, anger bias, and adults' different perceptions of Black and White children. *Cognition & Emotion*, *35*(7), 1416–1422. 10.1080/02699931.2021.1950127

Cosco, T. D., Fortuna, K., Wister, A., Riadi, I., Wagner, K., & Sixsmith, A. (2021). COVID-19, social isolation, and mental health among older adults: A digital catch-22. *Journal of Medical Internet Research*, *23*(5), e21864. 10.2196/21864

Feagin, J., & Bennefield, Z. (2014). Systemic racism and U.S. health care. *Social Science & Medicine (1982)*, *103*, 7–14. 10.1016/j.socscimed.2013.09.006

Goff, P. A., Jackson, M. C., Di Leone, B. A. L., Culotta, C. M., & DiTomasso, N. A. (2014). The essence of innocence: Consequences of dehumanizing Black children. *Journal of Personality and Social Psychology*, *106*(4), 526–545. 10.1037/a0035663

Healthy People 2030, U.S. Department of Health and Human Services, Office of Disease Prevention and Health Promotion. Retrieved [date graphic was accessed], from https://health.gov/healthypeople/objectives-and-data/social-determinants-health

Hoffman, K. M., Trawalter, S., Axt, J. R., & Oliver, M. N. (2016). Racial bias in pain assessment and treatment recommendations, and false beliefs about biological differences between Blacks and Whites. *PNAS Proceedings of the National Academy of Sciences of the United States of America, 113*(16), 4296–4301. 10.1073/pnas.1516047113

Sobalvarro, S. S., Cepeda, J. A., Garcia, J. T., Jackson, C., Shiang, E., Chakravarti, S., Workman, J., & Reese, J. M. (2023). The impact of COVID-19 on emotional, social, and behavioral health in adolescents with preexisting mental health concerns: A qualitative study. *Clinical Practice in Pediatric Psychology, 11*(2), 228–238. 10.1037/cpp0000485

Tomlin, J., & Völlm, B. (Eds.). (2022). *Diversity and marginalisation in forensic mental health care* (1st ed.). Routledge. 10.4324/9781003184768

Trawalter, S., Todd, A. R., Baird, A. A., & Richeson, J. A. (2008). Attending to threat: Race-based patterns of selective attention. *Journal of Experimental Social Psychology, 44*(5), 1322–1327. 10.1016/j.jesp.2008.03.006

Wells, B. A., & Kavanaugh, A. (2022). The US criminal justice system: The experience of racially marginalized people. In *Diversity and marginalisation in forensic mental health care* (pp. 9–17). Taylor and Francis. 10.4324/9781003184768-3

Wilson, J. P., Hugenberg, K., & Rule, N. O. (2017). Racial bias in judgments of physical size and formidability: From size to threat. *Journal of Personality and Social Psychology, 113*(1), 59–80. 10.1037/pspi0000092

Yale Medicine. (2021, October 1). Racial inequities in treatments of addictive disorders. *Yale Medicine.* https://medicine.yale.edu/news-article/racial-inequities-in-treatments-of-addictive-disorders/

Zhen-Duan, J., Colombo, D., Cruz-Gonzalez, M. A., Hoyos, M., & Alvarez, K. (2023). Adverse childhood experiences and alcohol use and misuse: Testing the impact of traditional and expanded adverse childhood experiences among racially/ethnically diverse youth transitioning into adulthood. *Psychological Trauma: Theory, Research, Practice, and Policy, 15*(Suppl 1), S55–S64. 10.1037/tra0001458

Chapter 5

Substance Use Treatment

Current Practices

Community Programs

Community programs have been a key resource for people in substance use recovery. The programs provide unity, support, and accountability to people in recovery through meetings and information sharing. These meetings provide an opportunity for individuals to have a shared experience and offer the opportunity for connection that is free of judgment. The first formal recovery group developed was Alcoholics Anonymous (AA). Heavily influenced by the Christian movement called "The Oxford Group," AA was founded shortly after the end of prohibition by Bill Wilson and Dr. Robert Smith in 1935. AA has expanded and evolved over the years to be seen as more inclusive. Due to its initial origins in Christianity, many individuals found themselves not being able to obtain the judgment-free connection they were seeking when in AA meetings. Additionally, individuals who did not have a religious background did not agree with some initial concepts proposed by AA. The main concept that God was in control and individuals seeking recovery needed to surrender to God was not well received by individuals of different spiritual backgrounds. Now, less of an emphasis is placed on Christianity explicitly, and AA utilizes a "higher power" as a concept instead of God specifically. However, many other community programs have been developed to meet the ever-changing needs of people in recovery. Below, you will be introduced to several community meetings that have formed since AA. This is not an exhaustive list, nonetheless the variety of community meetings and groups that have come about since AA shows the need for continued diversity in this area. It also shows a desire for, and benefit from, community connection and having a shared experience that brings people together. There are many unique benefits of these meetings as they pertain to cultural responsiveness. Knowing about the range of community meetings that exist is essential to providing culturally responsive substance use treatment as

DOI: 10.4324/9781032708829-5

well because one size does not fit all when participating in community meetings. By the time you finish this chapter, you will be able to provide clients with valuable recovery community programs that align with their unique cultural identities.

12-Step

12-Step programs are derivatives of AA. The term "12-Step" refers to the 12 steps that people in recovery are supposed to go through when they decide to participate in one of the programs. These steps are intended to contribute to an individual's journey to sobriety through various activities and perspectives that the steps encourage (Alcoholics Anonymous, n.d.). These programs include but are not limited to Narcotics Anonymous (NA), Cocaine Anonymous (CA), Crystal Meth Anonymous (CMA), Sexual Compulsives Anonymous (SCA), and Gamblers Anonymous (GA). Under the 12-Step umbrella, there are also meetings for those who are impacted in some way by a friend or loved one who is in an active addiction. These meetings include Codependents Anonymous (CODA), Al-Anon, and Alateen. These are just a few examples of many meetings and groups that serve the purpose of helping those impacted by friends or loved ones who have an active substance use disorder. Al-Anon and Alateen are specifically intended for people who have been impacted by a friend or loved one's drinking, but people impacted by a friend or loved one's substance use other than alcohol are not excluded from participation. The "Al" in Al-Anon and Alateen represent the "alcoholics" in "Alcoholics Anonymous." It is important to note that the terms "codependent" and "alcoholics" are not culturally responsive in that they do not utilize person-first language. They are also perceived as negative and carry value-laden depictions of individuals who have substance use disorders that are not accurate. In most cases, professionally, it is not appropriate to refer to an individual as an "alcoholic" or "codependent." There are several core tenets of 12-Step programs for people seeking recovery, however, the actual "steps" of 12-Step programs are the following:

1 Admitting powerlessness over the addiction
2 Believing that a higher power (in whatever form) can help
3 Deciding to turn control over to the higher power
4 Taking a personal inventory
5 Admitting to the higher power, oneself, and another person the wrongs done
6 Being ready to have the higher power correct any shortcomings in one's character
7 Asking the higher power to remove those shortcomings

8 Making a list of wrongs done to others and being willing to make amends for those wrongs
9 Contacting those who have been hurt, unless doing so would harm the person
10 Continuing to take personal inventory and admitting when one is wrong
11 Seeking enlightenment and connection with the higher power via prayer and meditation
12 Carrying the message of the 12 Steps to others in need

As noted, there is a heavy emphasis on a higher power and submitting to the higher power in some capacity. These steps are also accompanied by "The Big Book" which goes into more detail about each step, as well as recovery for those who participate in 12-Step programs. While the emphasis on relinquishing control to a higher power can be very liberating and supportive of recovery for some, others have a hard time understanding or engaging in some of the steps due to their own different religious or spiritual backgrounds. Additionally, those who do not believe in any form of a higher power are often left feeling like this is not the community for them or feel as though they are "faking" to get through their addiction.

The principles for programs dedicated to people impacted by one's substance use (Al-Anon and Alateen for example) are slightly different but still follow the 12-Step model. These programs also have traditions, promises, and service concepts that they introduce to those impacted by a friend or loved one's addiction. Below are the CoDA 12-Steps that are adapted from the AA 12-Steps to meet the needs of these individuals:

1 We admitted we were powerless over others – that our lives had become unmanageable.
2 Came to believe that a power greater than ourselves could restore us to sanity.
3 Made a decision to turn our will and our lives over to the care of God as we understood God.
4 Made a searching and fearless moral inventory of ourselves.
5 Admitted to God, to ourselves, and to another human being the exact nature of our wrongs.
6 Were entirely ready to have God remove all these defects of character.
7 Humbly asked God to remove our shortcomings.
8 Made a list of all persons we had harmed, and became willing to make amends to them all.
9 Made direct amends to such people wherever possible, except when to do so would injure them or others.

10 Continued to take personal inventory and when we were wrong promptly admitted it.
11 Sought through prayer and meditation to improve our conscious contact with God as we understood God, praying only for knowledge of God's will for us and the power to carry that out.
12 Having had a spiritual awakening as the result of these steps, we tried to carry this message to other codependents, and to practice these principles in all our affairs.

One thing to recognize is that CoDA does still use God within the 12-Steps outlined, which can be unrelatable to people with different spiritual backgrounds and those who do not identify with any spiritual or religious belief system.

Celebrate Recovery

As noted, AA was heavily influenced by Christianity when it was initially formed, however, as more people seeking recovery noted their discomfort with the heavy emphasis, AA shifted to utilizing the concept of a higher power instead of God specifically. Unfortunately, for those individuals who did identify as Christian, this shift was uncomfortable and no longer aligned with their spiritual or religious identity. As a result, Celebrate Recovery was formed. Like AA, Celebrate Recovery was developed to help individuals with various forms of addiction as well as "life issues." Formed in Saddleback Church located in Lake Forest, a city within Orange County of Southern California in 1991, John Baker and Pastor Rick Warren developed a Christ-centered recovery program for people to use for healing and freedom. Celebrate Recovery utilizes the 12-Steps from AA as a companion to bible verses that support each individual step. There is an explicit integration of biblical principles and ideals that are used to maintain the Christian aspect of the community program. An example of this is that all groups are gender specific. Celebrate Recovery meetings are hosted at church campuses and are marketed to a broad set of categories in which people struggle. As with AA, Celebrate Recovery is intended to build community and support with a Christian lens. Celebrate Recovery has expanded their program offerings to youth, Veterans, and what they identify as "cultural communities" to meet the needs of specific populations. Overall, the program follows a set of core principles that are intended to serve as a guide for individuals who are actively participating in Celebrate Recovery. These principles are the following:

1 Biblical Foundation: Celebrate Recovery is firmly grounded in biblical teachings and acknowledges Jesus Christ as the ultimate higher power who can bring restoration and recovery.

2   Acceptance: It emphasizes the importance of creating a safe and non-judgmental environment where people can openly share their struggles and find acceptance.
3   Transformation: The program seeks to promote personal transformation by encouraging individuals to surrender their problems to God, work through the steps, and experience spiritual growth.
4   Twelve Steps and Biblical Comparisons: Celebrate Recovery adopts the 12-Steps and combines them with corresponding biblical principles, creating a Christ-centered approach to recovery.
5   Small Groups: The program operates through small, gender-specific support groups where individuals can share their experiences, receive encouragement, and be held accountable in a confidential setting.
6   Step Studies: Step Studies are in-depth, gender-specific groups that explore the 12-Steps and corresponding biblical comparisons. These studies provide a more focused and structured approach to working through the recovery process.
7   Sponsorship: Celebrate Recovery encourages participants to seek out sponsors, individuals who have found healing in their own recovery journey, to provide support, guidance, and accountability.
8   Cross-Issues: The program recognizes that addiction and other life issues are often intertwined, and it offers specific resources and groups to address issues such as co-dependency, abuse, anger, and more.
9   Grace and Forgiveness: Celebrate Recovery emphasizes the power of grace and forgiveness in healing relationships and overcoming past hurts. It encourages participants to seek reconciliation with others and develop a deeper relationship with God.

Celebrate Recovery has had much success as an alternative to AA in part due to its clear "identity." Celebrate Recovery as a community program does not sugar-coat its Christ-centered focus, and individuals for which Christianity is a dominant part of their identity benefit from that clear designation. Additionally, those who participate in Celebrate Recovery are generally already connected to the church offering the program, which can be helpful for reducing fear about connecting with others. People who already belong to the church have an established relationship with other church members, making the connection aspect of community meetings less daunting.

Refuge Recovery

As mentioned, AA began to evolve and transition from using God specifically to a more general higher power. The goal here was to expand participation and more adequately meet the needs of individuals who wanted to participate in community support recovery programs. Still, this was not sufficient for individuals whose spiritual background did not align with the 12-Step principles. Celebrate Recovery was specific to people who identified as Christian and were in alignment with the principles outlined by Celebrate Recovery. The limitations of these community programs created a need that was seemingly filled by Refuge Recovery. Refuge Recovery was founded in 2014, by a meditation teacher named Noah Levine. Noah followed Buddhist principles and used them in his own recovery. He created Refuge Recovery as a Buddhist-inspired approach to recovery, focusing on healing and liberation (Refuge Recovery, n.d.). The development of Refuge Recovery was beneficial because it provided an alternative to Christian and Christian-light approaches to recovery. It also introduced alternative spiritual practices for individuals who did not ascribe to the concept of a higher power.

Refuge Recovery utilized two concepts central to Buddhism and adapted them to meet the specific needs of people who have an addiction. The concepts are known as the Four Noble Truths and the Noble Eightfold Path. Additionally, Refuge Recovery notes meditation as the "cornerstone" of the recovery path. These three concepts together are labeled as "The Buddhist System" in Refuge Recovery.

The Four Truths outlined by Refuge Recovery are as follows:

1st Truth: Addiction Creates Suffering; We take stock of all the suffering we have experienced and caused as addicts.

2nd Truth: The Cause of Addiction Is Repetitive Craving; We investigate the causes and conditions that lead to addiction and begin the process of letting go.

3rd Truth: Recovery is possible; We come to understand that recovery is possible and take refuge in the path that leads to the end of addiction.

4th Truth: The path to recovery is available; We engage in the process of the Eightfold Path that leads to recovery.

The Eightfold Path is considered the process that individuals go through that leads to recovery and includes the following:

1 Understanding
2 Intentions
3 Speech/community
4 Actions
5 Livelihood/service
6 Effort
7 Mindfulness
8 Concentration

Refuge Recovery, unlike AA or Celebrate Recovery, does not utilize a 12-Step model for their program but instead, adopts the Eightfold Path to guide recovery. It is also important to note that there is a consistent use of terms like "addict" in this community recovery program. This language is pervasive in the recovery community and prompts individuals to adopt "addict" as an identity to participate in these recovery communities.

The final, and most explicit aspect of Refuge Recovery is meditation. Refuge Recovery programs indicate that wisdom arises through the formal practice of mindful meditation. This wisdom allows individuals to see clearly and thus heal root causes that lead to "suffering of addiction." Specifically, mindfulness meditations, heart practice meditations, and forgiveness meditations are encouraged through Refuge Recovery throughout the entire recovery "path." Refuge Recovery can be a beneficial alternative to the previously mentioned community-based meetings as a supplemental form of support for individuals in recovery due to its nontheistic approach. Unlike AA or Celebrate Recovery, Refuge Recovery does not rely on the belief in a higher power or deity. Though there are principles that allude to power beyond consciousness, this power or control comes from within. Refuge Recovery encourages individuals to develop their own spiritual connection through meditation, mindfulness, and living in awareness.

Refuge Recovery is also appealing to individuals seeking community connection in recovery due to its openness to individuals from various backgrounds, including those with different religious or spiritual beliefs. There is no specific belief required to participate in Refuge Recovery, but there is a strong emphasis on the need for someone to develop competence in controlling their own behavior and taking ownership of their decisions. Additionally, the program highlights the varying impacts that addiction has on all aspects of life. Refuge Recovery integrates physical, mental, emotional, and spiritual wellness into its concepts. This results in Refuge Recovery encouraging a holistic approach to recovery, addressing the well-being of the whole person through meditation, self-inquiry, and "ethical living." The concept of "ethical living" is subjective, however, it is one aspect of this community recovery program that easily differentiates Refuge Recovery from other recovery programs. Ethical living is defined by Refuge Recovery as focusing on personal responsibility and ethical conduct as it pertains to an individual's substance use behavior. Overall, by integrating these teachings with personal experience and peer support, Refuge Recovery provides individuals with a self-directed framework for addressing their addiction and cultivating a life of compassion, wisdom, and sobriety.

SMART Recovery

SMART Recovery stands for "Self-Management and Recovery Training" and positions itself as a science-based, self-help program designed to assist individuals in overcoming various addictions and problematic behaviors (SMART Recovery, n.d.). SMART Recovery was founded in 1994 by Joe Gerstein, a medical doctor, and Tom Horvath, a clinical psychologist. SMART Recovery is another alternative to faith-based community recovery programs. The founders of SMART Recovery utilized principles from Cognitive Behavioral Therapy to develop a community program rooted in evidence-based practices for behavior change. SMART Recovery's emphasis is on behavior change. As such, there are modules, homework, and psychoeducation that accompany the program. SMART Recovery was a welcomed addition to community recovery programs for individuals who did not feel connected to or in alignment with spiritual or faith-based practices that accompanied AA or Celebrate Recovery. Additionally, Refuge Recovery had not yet been developed.

"Self-empowerment" instead of "admitting powerlessness" is one of SMART Recovery's core beliefs as it pertains to achieving recovery. The program places a strong emphasis on personal empowerment and self-reliance. Unlike other community recovery programs, it encourages participants to take control of their recovery journey and make informed decisions based on their own values and goals. SMART Recovery assists individuals in taking control through behavioral interventions adapted from scientific research and evidence-based practices. These practices come from psychological orientations such as cognitive-behavioral therapy (CBT), rational emotive behavior therapy (REBT), and motivational interviewing (MI). REBT focuses on identifying and challenging what they label as "irrational" beliefs and replacing them with healthier and more constructive thoughts and behaviors. The program emphasizes the importance of developing effective coping strategies, problem-solving skills, and emotional regulation techniques to assist in the recovery process. These interventions are intended to provide practical tools and resources to help individuals manage cravings, make choices that promote and maintain their recovery, and handle life's challenges.

These techniques and therapeutic interventions draw connections between thoughts, behaviors, and emotions to help individuals better understand why they engage in certain behaviors, as well as how thoughts and emotions impact the decision to engage in certain behaviors. SMART Recovery also recognizes that different individuals have diverse needs and preferences. This is illustrated through SMART Recovery having no requirement to follow a specific set of steps or beliefs. The program takes a more supportive approach to recovery by providing resources to help facilitate more adaptive decision-making strategies for the individual. This is displayed through a Four-Point Program that guides individuals through the recovery process. Though SMART Recovery is very explicit about the self-directed approach to recovery, these points are intended to help with guiding individuals to their own recovery. The points are: Building and Maintaining Motivation, Coping with Urges, Managing Thoughts, Feelings, and Behaviors, and Living a Balanced Life.

While SMART Recovery is a secular program, it welcomes participants from all backgrounds, including those with religious or spiritual beliefs. It does not incorporate a higher power concept or rely on spiritual principles but instead places emphasis on evidence-based practices, self-management, and choice. SMART Recovery has also expanded to offer programs specific to Veterans & First Responders, Young Adults, and people in the LGBTQIA+ community. As with other community programs listed, however, SMART Recovery has its own limitations that contribute to individuals not being able to feel connected to this community. SMART Recovery focuses very heavily on evidence-based practices, but these practices were developed and normed on predominantly White populations. These practices are very focused on the individual and do not consider systemic or societal barriers that contribute to one's addiction. There is also often an oversimplification of "irrational beliefs" and these beliefs of marginalized individuals tend to be mislabeled as "irrational" in SMART Recovery programs. Because of these limitations, racially marginalized individuals can develop unhealthy self-perceptions that are inaccurate or more harmful than helpful. This also leaves a gap for individuals who are seeking practical skills AND spiritual connection within their recovery journey. SMART Recovery is also a "solution-focused" approach to recovery in that the program does not take interest in the past, but instead, focuses on the future and how individuals can "move forward." This approach can be very helpful for some and provides individuals an opportunity to think about a healthy future. For others, much of their substance use is rooted in their past and they may need to address their past before feeling like they are able to adequately address their substance use.

Secular Organizations for Sobriety

In response to the initial emphasis in AA on a higher power and the need to admit powerlessness, Secular Organizations for Sobriety (SOS) was developed. SOS is also known as "Save Our Selves" and was founded by James Christopher. James was a former AA member and did not align with the spiritual component of AA. He founded SOS in 1985 to promote individuals taking personal responsibility for their sobriety, and to encourage individuals to identify what their own strengths and abilities were as they related to recovery. SOS has been branded as a "secular self-help alternative" to AA, and like SMART Recovery, SOS focuses on self-empowerment. Because it promotes the belief that individuals can overcome addiction through self-reliance and personal responsibility, the community recovery organization does not adhere to any specific religious or spiritual doctrine. The documentary "No God at the Bottom of a Glass" positioned SOS to become a more well-known community recovery group alternative to AA and provided individuals with recovery community options.

SOS as an organization believes that sobriety is a separate issue from everything else, and abstinence is "priority one, no matter what!" The general principles of SOS, which are outlined in the SOS brochure are the following:

- All those who sincerely seek sobriety are welcome as members in any SOS Group.
- SOS is not a spin-off of any religious or secular group. There is no hidden agenda, as SOS is concerned with achieving and maintaining sobriety (abstinence).
- SOS seeks only to promote sobriety amongst those who suffer from addictions. As a group, SOS has no opinion on outside matters and does not wish to become entangled in outside controversy.
- Although sobriety is an individual responsibility, life does not have to be faced alone. The support of other alcoholics and addicts is a vital adjunct to recovery. In SOS, members share experiences, insights, information, strength, and encouragement in friendly, honest, anonymous, and supportive group meetings.
- To avoid unnecessary entanglements, each SOS group is self-supporting through contributions from its members and refuses outside support.
- Sobriety is the number-one priority in a recovering person's life. As such, he or she must abstain from all drugs or alcohol.
- Honest, clear, and direct communication of feelings, thoughts, and knowledge aids in recovery and in choosing nondestructive, nondelusional, and rational approaches to living sober and rewarding lives.
- As knowledge of addiction might cause a person harm or embarrassment in the outside world, SOS guards the anonymity of its membership and the contents of its discussions from those not within the group.
- SOS encourages the scientific study of all aspects of alcoholism and addiction. SOS does not limit its outlook to one area of knowledge or theory of alcoholism and addiction.

As with many other community-based recovery programs, SOS holds group recovery meetings for individuals to connect with others in recovery.

Unlike the other organizations though, SOS does not have a specific set of principles outside of the general principles outlined above. There are no specific guidelines or "steps" in SOS, and the main priority of SOS is the concept of "sobriety priority," which involves making sobriety the primary focus in one's life and aligning one's choices and actions accordingly. SOS does not have meetings or programs catered to any specific demographic group, which can be helpful in contributing to feelings of connectedness. However, it also prevents SOS from meeting the unique needs of marginalized individuals.

Women for Sobriety

Women for Sobriety (WFS) was founded in 1975 by Jean Kirkpatrick, who was trained as a Sociologist. This community recovery program was developed by Kirkpatrick due to her observation of the need for a recovery program that catered to the specific experiences and issues faced by women who had an addiction. WFS has a "New Life" program as the core of their community recovery organization (Women for Sobriety, n.d.). Within that program, there are 13 "Acceptance Statements" that women are encouraged to read and reflect on each morning. The statements are as follows:

1 I have a life-threatening problem that once had me.
   I now take charge of my life and my well-being. I accept the responsibility.
2 Negative thoughts destroy only myself.
   My first conscious sober act is to reduce negativity in my life.
3 Happiness is a habit I am developing.
   Happiness is created, not waited for.
4 Problems bother me only to the degree I permit.
   I now better understand my problems. I do not permit problems to overwhelm me.
5 I am what I think.
   I am a capable, competent, caring, compassionate woman.
6 Life can be ordinary or it can be great.
   Greatness is mine by a conscious effort.
7 Love can change the course of my world.
   Caring is all-important.
8 The fundamental object of life is emotional and spiritual growth.
   Daily I put my life into a proper order, knowing which are the priorities.
9 The past is gone forever.
   No longer am I victimized by the past. I am a new woman.
10 All love given returns.
   I am learning to know that I am loved.

11 Enthusiasm is my daily exercise.
I treasure the moments of my New Life.
12 I am a competent woman, and I have much to give life.
This is what I am, and I shall know it always.
13 I am responsible for myself and for my actions.
I am in charge of my mind, my thoughts, and my life.

In addition to the 13 Acceptance Statements, there are six levels of recovery outlined in the WFS program that are paired with the Acceptance Statements. These levels of recovery are used in the program to promote self-reflection, and often are accompanied by journaling. The following are the levels outlined for the New Life Program:

Level 1 – Acceptance of having a substance use disorder, one that requires the cessation of substance use.

Level 2 – Discarding negative thoughts, putting guilt behind, and practicing new ways of viewing and solving problems.

Level 3 – Creating and practicing a new self-image.

Level 4 – Using new attitudes to enforce new behavior patterns.

Level 5 – Improving relationships as a result of our new feelings about self.

Level 6 – Recognizing life's priorities: emotional and spiritual growth, self-responsibility.

Although WFS also identifies as a secular organization, there is an emphasis on emotional and spiritual growth as part of their program and recovery process. The New Life program within WFS also encourages women to develop self-esteem, self-worth, and self-acceptance as they work toward sobriety. WFS is an organization that exhibits focus on self-love, self-discovery, and women's empowerment. What makes this community recovery program so unique is their gender-specific approach to recovery, and their explicit focus on addressing the unique needs and experiences of women.

The diversity of meetings is very beneficial for cultivating culturally responsive environments for people in recovery. Although this is not an exhaustive list, these community recovery organizations are attempting to meet the needs of individuals from *the identity of the individual*. There is a clear need for a diverse set of offerings from community recovery programs as a supplement to professional support. These community recovery programs also show that there are a wide range of community recovery program styles to choose from. Some are more structured, while others are fluid. Some programs follow spiritual principles and others are squarely focused on what is within one's control. The evolution and expansion of these community-led programs shows how valuable and needed culturally responsive substance use treatment is today. These programs will continue to expand to meet diverse individual needs, however, culture is ever-evolving, and identities continually change over time. The need for connection and community over shared experiences and identities will always be present. This is where self-help apps have stepped in.

Self-Help Apps

The community recovery meetings listed above do not cover all community recovery meetings that exist. The list does however show the variety of options for community meeting participation that are available to people in recovery. It is my hope that health care organizations and providers will make more of an effort to share information about different meetings instead of prioritizing AA. It is also my hope that organizations consider offering these types of meetings in their wellness packages for their staff.

In recent years, the landscape of community recovery meetings and programs has continued to experience an increased need to diversify their offerings. This need has contributed to the emergence of recovery-based self-help applications (apps). These digital platforms have provided individuals with new avenues for support and assistance in their journey towards recovery. They have increased the accessibility of and the definition of a recovery community for individuals who were seeking recovery but did not have access to the traditional recovery meeting. There has also been a notable increase in the adoption and traction of these apps, particularly in response to the challenges posed by the COVID-19 pandemic.

Recovery-based self-help apps operate on the premise of utilizing technology to extend support networks beyond the limitations of physical meetings. These apps typically offer a range of features designed to facilitate engagement, education, and connection within the recovery community. Some common functionalities include virtual meetings, progress tracking, educational resources, meditation and mindfulness exercises, peer support forums, and access to trained counselors or sponsors. The early iterations of recovery apps primarily focused on providing basic information and resources related to substance use disorders and recovery. However, as technology advanced and user feedback accumulated, these apps evolved to address the diverse needs and preferences of individuals seeking recovery. App developers recognized the importance of tailoring the user experience to different populations, considering factors such as age, gender, cultural background, and specific substance use issues. Some existing community recovery programs, SMART Recovery for example, have taken to the evolution of community recovery support by launching their own accompanying app to their program. The adoption of technology by existing community recovery programs has been expedited by the development of these recovery-based apps.

To meet the needs of diverse individuals, recovery apps have integrated personalized features and content. Users can set goals and preferences, enabling the app to curate relevant resources, meeting recommendations, and tailored support. These apps also employ strategies from evidence-based approaches, such as cognitive-behavioral therapy, motivational interviewing, and mindfulness-based practices, providing users with targeted interventions that align with their recovery goals. The advent of the COVID-19 pandemic created unprecedented challenges for the substance use recovery community. Social distancing measures, lockdowns, and the closure of in-person support meetings disrupted the traditional avenues of connection and support. In response, recovery-based self-help applications gained even more traction as a vital lifeline for individuals seeking recovery during these difficult times.

The pandemic accelerated the adoption of these apps, as they provided a means to maintain and enhance support networks while adhering to physical distancing guidelines. Virtual meetings became a staple feature of many recovery apps, allowing individuals to participate in group discussions, share experiences, and receive encouragement from peers, all from the safety and comfort of their own homes. The convenience and accessibility of recovery apps became paramount, enabling individuals to connect with support 24/7, regardless of their geographical location. Moreover, recovery apps adapted to the unique challenges of the pandemic by incorporating features specifically designed to address COVID-related concerns. For instance, some apps included sections dedicated to managing stress and anxiety related to the pandemic, offering resources and tools to cope with isolation, uncertainty, and triggers that may arise during these times.

Recovery-based self-help applications have undergone a remarkable evolution, catering to the diverse needs of individuals seeking support in their journey towards recovery. These apps have emerged as a valuable complement to traditional community recovery meetings and programs. The COVID-19 pandemic further propelled the adoption of these apps, as they offered a lifeline of connection, support, and resources during a time of unprecedented challenges. As technology continues to advance, it is anticipated that recovery apps will continue to innovate and refine their offerings, ensuring that they remain relevant and effective in supporting individuals on their path to recovery. As this happens, it will be important to continue ensuring cultural identity is in alignment with the types of apps used by people in recovery.

Treatment Approaches

Current treatment approaches to substance use that exist are well established in the professional community of addiction medicine providers. Unfortunately, the commonly used treatment approaches and addiction frameworks generally lack a culturally responsive foundation. Treatment approaches that do consider cultural factors are usually an adaptation of existing treatment modalities, which are rooted in non-culturally responsive concepts. Additionally, there is little agreement among providers and agencies serving the recovery community regarding best approach, which contributes to a lack of adequate care. Inconsistencies in treatment approaches hinder the retention of diverse individuals who are seeking treatment for substance use. Understanding the current treatment landscape, as well as the origins of the treatment approaches provides context for why culturally responsive substance use treatment is necessary for truly effective care.

Thombs and Osborn (2019) note explicitly their efforts to include cultural factors related to addiction in their fifth edition of Introduction to Addictive Behaviors. Although there have been previous editions of the book, it was not until 2019 that substance use stigma was covered in detail. Since this book is often used in substance use training programs as a foundational academic supplement for understanding treatment approaches, it is encouraging to know that efforts are being made to increase awareness of the sociocultural aspects of addiction. Still, there are limitations to the current reading material related to substance use treatment approaches. Namely, these existing treatment approaches were developed without consideration or attention to cultural uniqueness or cultural-historical factors. Additionally, many of these treatment approaches were developed by systems that perpetuate oppression. Couched as "evidence-based practices" the evidence base comes primarily from non-marginalized communities, begging the question that this is evidence-based, but for whom? Although there has been discussion regarding cultural competence in mental health treatment, there is also no motive for agencies to change their longstanding practices. Further, research to develop culturally responsive evidence-based practices is faced with challenge. Prestigious journals reject articles due to "lack of scientific merit" if they are primarily qualitative. Students of color and academics of color are covertly deterred from conducting research for minoritized communities with minoritized community samples. Proposals are rejected based on the history of publications without consideration for the systemic limitations of people of color who attempt to publish but are rejected for the reasons listed above. There are several factors that contribute to why culturally responsive evidence-based practices are not seeing the light of day, but it is not because the work is not being done; it is because the work is being hidden or pushed out due to the institutional practices that perpetuate oppression.

The Disease Model of Addiction

The Disease Model of Addiction, also known as the medical model, originated in the mid-20th century and was primarily influenced by Alcoholics Anonymous (AA). This model views addiction as a chronic, relapsing brain disease and most importantly, that substance use is a product of, rather than the root cause of addiction. This means addiction as a disease is that causes substance use, and the disease is uncurable. In the last decade, the medical profession has adapted its definition of addiction to remove the absolute nature of "disease" by adding that addiction is a "curable disease." However, this model heavily depends on medication to achieve abstinence and places a large emphasis on genetic factors contributing to an individual developing an addiction. The disease model emphasizes complete abstinence from substances as the primary goal of treatment and ascribes to the AA concept that an individual is powerless over their addiction.

Given the disease model's origins in medicine and its connection to AA principles, this model perpetuates the idea that individuals with substance use disorders are morally flawed. It also strongly aligns with an "all or nothing" approach to recovery that includes medication and admittance of loss of control by the individual. These foundational aspects of the disease model can lead to increased stigma and self-blame. The emphasis on abstinence as the sole treatment goal may not align with the preferences and goals of all individuals, particularly those who may experience more benefit from a harm reduction approach.

Psychoanalytic Approaches to Addiction Treatment

Psychoanalytic approaches to addiction treatment are adaptations of psychodynamic theories of psychology and mental health treatment. Heavily oriented in the exploration of unconscious conflicts, these theories have long been criticized for their lack of empirical support. However, since this theoretical orientation was introduced by one of the early "fathers" of psychology, Sigmund Freud, the lack of evidence base for this approach is often overlooked. As previously noted, having the label of evidence-based does not inherently mean the treatment approach is effective for all individuals, however, the complete lack or inconsistency of treatment outcomes is not the answer to developing effective and comprehensive treatment approaches either.

The psychoanalytic approach to substance use treatment is rooted in how the treatment provider interprets the information given by the individual in treatment. The information given by the person in treatment can come in various forms including dreams, free association, and the client's "resistance" to treatment. Additionally, how the treatment provider feels toward the client and vice versa (counter-transference and transference) also play a role in the treatment approach. One of the most salient concerns with this approach, as it pertains to cultural responsiveness, is the fact that all information is interpreted by another individual. This subjective technique ignores different lived experiences had by the treatment provider and the individual receiving treatment. Additionally, most psychoanalytic inter-pretations are rooted in the idea that the source of any issue originates from unconscious feelings toward primary caregivers from one's childhood. This source of interpretation lends itself to wrongful blaming of family members and ignores societal contributions to circumstances that require a child to be in a household with two working parents for example. There is benefit in exploring unconscious thoughts in treat-ment, but there needs to be a fundamental understanding of, and consideration for, the extenuating factors that contribute to an indivi-dual's substance use.

Cognitive Models of Addiction Treatment

Cognitive models of addiction treatment focus on the role of cognitive processes, thoughts, and beliefs in the development and maintenance of substance use disorders. Cognitive restructuring is a common interven-tion for use in addiction treatment, with emphasis placed on identifying and challenging irrational thoughts and beliefs related to substance use, which leads to the restructuring of those thoughts and beliefs to be more adaptive to an abstinent lifestyle. The focus in models specific to cognitive processes as they pertain to addiction is skill-building. These skill-building techniques, for example assertiveness training, are used in part due to the thought that an individual using substances is using because they lack skills to do something different.

This approach to substance use treatment can be helpful in that it focuses on thought processes and patterns to be changed for an individual to make different decisions regarding substance use. Unfortunately, cognitive models for addiction treatment do not consider the whole person. An individual's thoughts are labeled "distortions" if they are not in alignment with what predominantly Western and culture-dominant societies agree with. This alienates individuals who come from different cultural backgrounds and have perspectives that may be labeled "distortions" but are very normal and sometimes even protective in their communities. Additionally, cognitive models of addiction treatment are limited when considering co-occurring diagnoses. Considering social determinants of health, trauma, and systemic oppression are critical when conceptualizing an individual's thoughts and beliefs. The intersection of these issues and substance use is often not highlighted or addressed when approaching substance use treatment from a cognitive model. Cognitive models also place much of the responsibility on the individual through skill-building and cognitive restructuring interventions.

Behavioral Models of Addiction Treatment

Often behavioral models of addiction treatment are merged with cognitive models, but it is important to clarify that cognitive behavioral models of treatment are different from pure cognitive and pure behavioral models of treatment. While Cognitive Behavioral Therapy (CBT) is the integration of both treatment approaches, this section is focused on behavioral models because many community-based recovery programs emphasize behavior change as a core function of recovery. Behavioral models of addiction treatment focus on changing behavior patterns associated with substance use through behavioral learning principles and techniques. Contingency Management (CM) is a well-known and effective form of addiction treatment due to its immediate reinforcement of adaptive behaviors. For example, if a program utilized CM as an intervention for substance use treatment, it would look like program participants receiving a monetary reward every time they submitted an undetected drug test. This immediate reward serves as a reinforcement strategy to encourage and maintain desired changes. CM is a purely behavioral approach that utilizes tangible rewards or incentives to reinforce positive behaviors, such as abstinence or treatment adherence. An additional component of CM is that it often employs a token economy system where individuals earn tokens for desired behaviors, which can be exchanged for rewards or privileges. This provides immediate reward in the form of a token, as well as delayed reinforcement because the tokens can be collected to exchange for larger or more desirable prizes.

Behavioral models have their limitations regarding cultural responsiveness. Often the overemphasis on behaviors is invalidating and dismissive of the experiences diverse individuals have, leaving them to feel as though the addiction is solely based on their behaviors. This is inaccurate and can be harmful to an individual in recovery. There is an association made between the behavior and the incentive within treatment, but outside of treatment, the incentive is either diminished, delayed, or non-existent. This prevents the behavioral changes within treatment from generalizing to outside of treatment. In addition to the lack of generalizability with behavioral models of substance use treatment, like the cognitive models, skills training focuses on the individual and often underemphasizes other psychological, social, or environmental factors that contribute to the behavior to being with. Although skills training is beneficial, it only addresses a portion of substance use treatment which in itself is a limitation.

Family System Models of Addiction Treatment

Family system models of addiction treatment view addiction as a function of family dynamics, identifying roles family members play in an individual's development, maintenance, and recovery from addiction. In many of these models, there is still an "identified patient" within the family system, who is generally the person using the substances, however, each family member develops a "role" in response to the identified patient's substance use. The idea is that a need is not being met for each person in the family system due to the identified patient's substance use and for the family to be balanced or achieve "homeostasis" each family member engages in their own maladaptive behavior. As a result of the unmet need and attempt to achieve homeostasis, other family members attempt to behave differently within their family system. An example of this would be if a parent were using substances and the substance use prevented the parent from attending their child's sporting activities. The other parent might engage in the behavior of lying on behalf of the other parent to spare the child's feelings. The child might perceive the parent who uses substances is not proud and try harder to gain the parent's attention. The sibling might step in to help the parent who does not use substances to reduce the burden observed.

This is just one example of how addiction is conceptualized from a family systems model. As with the conceptualization, substance use treatment from a family systems approach includes the participation of family members in therapy sessions, aiming to improve communication, address conflicts, and enhance support for the individual seeking treatment by involving family members in the process. In family systems treatment of addiction, there is a clear intersection between familial relationships and substance use that is targeted and addressed in treatment. Unfortunately, for minoritized and marginalized individuals, the framework of "family" may not match the treatment framework, leaving individuals from these backgrounds to feel as though something is "wrong" with their family. The framework also limits treatment from a systemic perspective because individuals who consider family members who are not blood-related are not able to bring those "chosen" family members into treatment due to legal limitations.

Motivational Theories of Addiction Treatment

Motivational Interviewing (MI) is more of an intervention for substance use treatment rather than a theory, however, there is a conceptual framework from which MI is derived which is person-centered theory. The idea that the client is the expert and can come to their own conclusions with openness and guidance from their therapist is what drives much of this approach. MI focuses on enhancing an individual's intrinsic motivation to change their substance use behaviors through Open-ended questioning, affirming, reflecting, and summarizing (OARS) (Miller & Rollnick, 2013). This approach emphasizes collaboration, empathy, and evoking individuals' own reasons for change. MI also posits that an individual who has a substance use condition is likely ambivalent about their substance use and uses MI as an approach to facilitate "change talk" in the individual as it pertains to their relationship with substances.

Motivational approaches to addiction treatment heavily emphasize "change" and one's desire to "change" when discussing substance use. This perspective eliminates the role of systems and power that impact minoritized and marginalized individuals who have substance use conditions. Like behavioral approaches to addiction treatment, this perspective can be extremely invalidating and ignores societal issues that contribute to substance use in these communities. Additionally, this approach tends to facilitate a way of thinking about individuals with substance use conditions as having ambivalence to their substance use and diminishes the role of environment, psychological distress, and culture.

Public Health Approaches to Addiction Treatment

Public health approaches to addiction treatment have evolved in response to the recognition of substance use as a public health issue. For example, SAMHSA has endorsed evidence-based techniques such as Community Reinforcement and Family Training (CRAFT) and the Adolescent Community Reinforcement approach (A-CRA) to provide more culturally appropriate substance use treatment to adults and adolescents. Both models make attempts to incorporate the community into treatment through the linkage of programs and cross-utilization of public health department offerings. Additionally, public health approaches are of the few approaches to embrace harm-reduction strategies as interventions for addiction treatment. Recognizing that abstinence-only can serve as a barrier to accomplishing the goal of improving public health, these approaches recognize that abstinence may not be an immediate or realistic goal for people who have substance use conditions. Public health approaches are also unique in their emphasis on educating the public and increasing awareness of substance use conditions, incorporating prevention programs as a key part of the approach.

Though public health approaches are more encompassing of outreach and community engagement, access to treatment and services offered is still a limitation in public health approaches. Trainings for CRAFT and A-CRA can be expensive, limiting the number of providers qualified to deliver these specific services, and limited providers leads to limited access to care. Additionally, outreach activities and prevention education is not encompassing of the marginalized and minoritized communities disproportionately impacted by substance use. Given that the public health approach also focuses on intervention at the population-level, unique needs of individuals historically not represented in the population are not benefiting from the approach.

Sociocultural Approaches to Addiction Treatment

As mentioned, sociocultural approaches to addiction treatment have also gained more traction in recent years. The five overlapping sociocultural functions of substance use are social facilitation, release from social obligations, repudiation of social norms, marking boundaries, and crossing boundaries. These concepts represent overarching commonalities in cultures regarding the reason for substance use, from building social connections to going against social norms. These approaches allow providers to understand the origins of substance use from a variety of perspectives and encourage an understanding of the client's values.

Note that there are little to no practical interventions to this approach. It takes into consideration one's possible reason for substance use, but it does not provide ways to address substance use. Instead, it provides a sociological perspective and explanation for substance use. Thombs and Osborn (2019) note that the lack of practicality in this approach will keep it from gaining status in the profession.

It is important to note that there is information out there on how to develop culturally competent mental health practices. Unfortunately, they are often not utilized for substance use treatment. There needs to be an explicit overhaul of existing practices, the status quo of substance use treatment, and an understanding that culture is an evolutionary concept, which means treatment should evolve with culture. Additionally, this concept of evolving treatment goes hand in hand with the difference between competence and responsiveness. Cultural competence assumes once an individual is trained in an area or an agency obtains certification in a treatment approach, there is no need to adapt and grow. Truthfully, agencies need to be *responsive* to their client populations and obtain a fluid approach to engaging in substance use treatment. It needs to be flexible enough to meet the needs of any individual who comes in the door and structured enough to be adopted at a system level. While each of these treatment approaches has its unique components and benefits, it is crucial to acknowledge their limitations in meeting the needs of diverse individuals. Cultural relevance, individualized care, and sensitivity to systemic factors are essential considerations in developing more comprehensive and inclusive substance use treatment approaches that address the diverse needs and experiences of individuals seeking help for addiction. The next portion of this book will discuss how this can be achieved.

References

Alcoholics Anonymous. (n.d.). *Alcoholics Anonymous.* https://www.aa.org/

Celebrate Recovery. (n.d.). *Celebrate Recovery.* https://www.celebraterecovery.com/

Miller, W. R. , & Rollnick, S. (2013). *Motivational interviewing: Helping people change* (3rd ed.). The Guilford Press.

Refuge Recovery. (n.d.). *Refuge Recovery.* https://www.refugerecovery.org/

SMART Recovery. (n.d.). *SMART Recovery.* https://www.smartrecovery.org/

SOS Sobriety. (n.d.). *SOS Sobriety.* https://www.sossobriety.org/

Thombs, D. L., & Osborn, C. J. (2019). *Introduction to addictive behaviors* (5th ed.). The Guilford Press.

Women for Sobriety. (n.d.). *Women for Sobriety.* https://womenforsobriety.org/

Chapter 6

BJED&I in Mental Health
The Copy Paste Method of Equity

The title of this chapter is important to discuss. What is not addressed when engaging in conversations about mental health and substance use treatment is that, oftentimes, whenever the mental health profession becomes "aware" of an issue and begins to address it, the substance use profession simply copies the approach taken within the context of mental health. Very little consideration for the nuance of having a substance use condition or having co-occurring conditions is taken. Furthermore, even with the developing understanding of the "co-occurring" concept, many mental health agencies and providers will not provide mental health services to individuals if substance use is present. One example of how substance use treatment has historically followed mental health but may not be effective is the approach to prescribing medication. In the profession of mental health, medication is often a common and well-accepted intervention used to manage symptoms of psychiatric conditions such as depression or anxiety. However, when it comes to substance use conditions, the use of medications can be more complex and require a different approach.

For instance, let's consider the case of a person with both a substance use condition and who has been diagnosed with depression. In the mental health profession, it might be common to prescribe an antidepressant medication to address the depressive symptoms. However, in the substance use profession, simply prescribing antidepressants without considering the substance use can be ineffective and potentially risky. Substances such as alcohol or certain other non-prescribed substances can interact with medications, leading to adverse effects or reduced effectiveness. Moreover, some medications used to treat mental health conditions, for example, benzodiazepines, can have addictive properties themselves and can exacerbate substance use disorders. Furthermore, they can contribute to the development of a substance use disorder.

In this example, a more effective approach would be to consider the interaction between the individual's substance use and their mental

DOI: 10.4324/9781032708829-6

health condition. Instead of solely relying on medication, an integrated treatment plan would address both the substance use and the mental health aspects concurrently. This may involve utilizing specialized substance use interventions such as motivational interviewing or contingency management in addition to medication. It may mean utilizing more holistic approaches before introducing medication as a treatment intervention. By tailoring the treatment to the unique challenges and needs of individuals with co-occurring substance use and mental health conditions, a more comprehensive and effective approach can be achieved.

It's essential for the substance use profession to recognize the nuances and complexities of treating substance use disorders, rather than simply adopting interventions developed solely within the context of mental health. When discussing the concept of Belonging, Justice, Equity, Diversity, and Inclusion (BJED&I), there are several ways in which the mental health profession has attempted to increase societal awareness of mental health conditions, destigmatize mental health conditions, and encourage individuals to seek treatment for mental health conditions without fear of judgment or discrimination. The same cannot be said for substance use treatment, and the same approach cannot be directly applied to substance use. There is a significant stigma that still surrounds substance use and substance use treatment. This stigma creates unique challenges in implementing effective Equity, Diversity, & Inclusion (ED&I) efforts in the substance use profession. Substance use disorders have long been associated with moral failings, criminality, and personal weaknesses, leading to a deeply ingrained societal stigma. This stigma is perpetuated by various factors, including media portrayals, societal attitudes, and historical criminalization of drug use. As a result, individuals with substance use disorders often face discrimination, social exclusion, and limited access to healthcare resources.

In a study conducted by Yang et al. (2017), researchers found that substance use disorders were more stigmatized than mental health disorders. The study revealed that society held more negative attitudes towards individuals with substance use disorders, often driven by stereotypes, discrimination, and having negative emotional reactions toward people with substance use conditions. The Johns Hopkins School of Public Health conducted a study published in 2014 also showing that the public continues to label individuals with substance use disorders as personally responsible for their condition compared to individuals with mental health disorders. This perception is framed as a "moral failing" of individuals with substance use conditions but is less so for individuals with mental health conditions. Due to this persistent stigma, efforts to increase EDI in substance use treatment must address and challenge societal attitudes and stereotypes surrounding substance use. Simply using the same framework utilized for mental health conditions to reduce stigma is not sufficient. It requires a multi-faceted approach that goes beyond solely destigmatizing the individuals seeking treatment but also targets the wider public perception of substance use disorders. Here's an example to illustrate the disparity between mental health and substance use in terms of EDI.

A mental health clinic has made conscious attempts to implement EDI efforts by hiring individuals from varying cultural backgrounds with diverse identities and creating a welcoming environment for clients from various backgrounds through signage and program offerings. The clinic actively promotes the message that seeking mental health treatment is a courageous and positive step towards personal well-being for their staff and clients. Clients are encouraged to openly discuss their mental health issues, and the stigma associated with mental health is gradually diminished. However, in the substance use treatment center within the same clinic, clients receiving services are met with assumptions from their providers that they are engaging in "help-seeking behaviors" are being "manipulative." They experience a sense of mistrust from their providers due to the program's heavy focus on "days sober" and barrier to obtaining mental health services until the client receives a "clean drug test." The signage as it pertains to substance use often reflects someone who appears to have not showered, is unhoused, and is in significant emotional distress.

This example highlights the need to understand BJED&I within the context of substance use treatment issues instead of simply "copying and pasting" the models used for mental health treatment that facilitate an increase in BJED&I in the mental health profession. Substance use treatment organizations must go beyond surface-level diversity for their staff. This can look like eliminating discriminatory hiring practices that disproportionately penalize individuals with substance use histories and consider an individual's qualifications, experience, recovery status, and commitment to personal growth when evaluating their suitability for positions within the profession. From a client's perspective, this can look like increasing access to varying models of treatment focused more on wellness and recovery and less on "days sober" or perceived maladaptive behaviors. Imagery reflecting individuals in recovery obtaining life-saving medication such as Narcan can promote an environment of hope and healing for clients. The concept of how BJED&I is being implemented in mental health and copied onto substance use without consideration of unique differences continues to perpetuate the need for a more culturally responsive and comprehensive approach to equity in substance use treatment.

Person-First Language

From a client's perspective, "Addict" can be a term that many people in recovery take pride in. People who refer to themselves as "addict" with pride generally have participated in Alcoholics Anonymous (AA), an affiliate Anonymous group, or other community-based recovery program. Several community-based recovery programs use the term "addict" to promote individuals "taking ownership" of their substance use to begin engagement of the recovery process. These programs utilize "addict" to describe individuals who participate in the programs and in their resource materials for the programs. It is a widespread term in the recovery community and is frequently used as a descriptor in conversations among treatment professionals and clients alike. In several other cases though, this label elicits shame, guilt, or blame if used to describe someone else. The mental health profession has attempted to increase equity and reduce stigma through the encouragement to use person-first language, that is, refer to the person, and then identify what behavior in which they engage. An example of this would be, "person with anxiety."

However, person-first language is still not utilized consistently when discussing substance use, and the person-first concept is actively rejected by some substance use professionals. Dunn and Andrews (2015) provided context supporting the notion that utilizing person-first language increases cultural competence in mental health providers. Baker et al.'s (2022) research confirmed that the use of post-modified nouns (person-first) in substance use treatment were associated with less stigmatizing and more benevolent attitudes toward people who use substances than the use of pre-modified (behavior-first) nouns. Even with the knowledge of how person-first language can be beneficial in reducing stigma, professionals in the substance use treatment community do not consistently utilize this approach to how they describe individuals with substance use conditions. Examples of how this concept is used for addiction include "a person with a substance use disorder," or "a person who uses substances." The utilization of person-first language is only half of the puzzle when implementing this concept into the substance use profession. What is not adequately addressed in use of person-first language for substance use treatment is the history of the term "addict" and the value placed on the term by individuals in recovery. It is unique in that "addict" can be perceived as a term of empowerment, whereas for a general mental health condition, schizophrenia for example, calling someone "a schizophrenic" doesn't carry an empowering message to anyone. Though person-first language is tremendously valuable for reducing stigma in the substance use community, there needs to be attention paid to how to accomplish the adoption of person-first language keeping cultural responsiveness in mind.

It is essential to consider the potential challenges and limitations of implementing person-first language without understanding cultural nuances. Simply eradicating the term without understanding its cultural significance could alienate those who find empowerment or solidarity in the label. This is not to say the term "addict" should continue being used, instead it is an invitation to expand the identities of an individual in recovery to reflect themselves more holistically. When describing culture, oftentimes "Recovery Lifestyle" is not included, but as we work toward equity in treatment of individuals with substance use conditions, Recovery Lifestyle is one of the first things to consider as we integrate person-first language in substance use treatment. Recovery culture is informed by one's individual identities, the relationship individuals have to their substance and substance use, and their perception of substance use from a combination of their experiences and societal influences.

Recovery culture can be illustrated through the example of Joseph. Joseph recently decided to seek treatment for his cannabis use. Joseph uses he/them pronouns, identifies as Indigenous, belongs to a gym, is part of "Gen Z," and serves as primary caregiver for his mother. He has two dogs and enjoys being outdoors. Prior to seeking treatment, Joseph participated in a community-based recovery program that emphasized "addict" as a preferred term to describe individuals in the program. Joseph initially experienced discomfort with identifying himself as an "addict" in part due to his relationship with substances. Joseph was introduced to cannabis early in life, as a plant in nature used for several medicinal purposes. Joseph has experienced friends and relatives utilize cannabis in various ways, and his mother uses cannabis to assist with her chronic pain.

In Joseph's community, various forms of plant medicine have also been crucial to his Indigenous identity and beliefs. He has seen the way cannabis use is portrayed in the media and does not identify with the stereotype that he doesn't take care of himself physically, but he began attending recovery meetings because Joseph wanted to explore alternative ways to "loosen up" his muscles post workout and believed he may have been using cannabis too frequently to accomplish this goal. When he began attending the recovery meetings, he obtained resources about being an "addict" and eventually adopted the concept believing there was no alternative. When Joseph entered treatment, it was related to his "sober curiosity." He completely abstained from cannabis while participating in the community program out of respect for the process, but Joseph was curious to know if there was another way.

By the time Joseph entered treatment, they had adopted the "addict" identity. They had become very hard on themselves when even thinking of cannabis, which promoted feelings of shame and guilt. Joseph also shared with their mother that she "needed to stop" using cannabis or Joseph would no longer be able to serve as their mother's caregiver. Joseph's Recovery Lifestyle became harmful to his other identities, but he had trouble seeing himself as anything other than an "addict." A part of him was proud that he was able to abstain from cannabis, but another part of him began drifting away from identities he cherished. He found himself avoiding aspects of his Indigenous background, not being a helpful caregiver to his mother, and experiencing personal shame and guilt for continuing to have thoughts about using cannabis on occasion.

In this example, although Joseph has adopted the identity "addict" because of his experience in the community recovery program, he has lost much of his other identities in the process. Helping an individual who has a substance use condition from the perspective of helping them develop their own Recovery Lifestyle provides a culturally responsive foundation in the substance use treatment approach. This includes providing psychoeducation about person-first language and acknowledging the historical value placed on language in the substance use community that is not person-first. It is crucial to engage in collaborative and culturally sensitive conversations with individuals and communities to ensure that person-first language is implemented appropriately, respectfully, and approved by the client.

The benefits of person-first language in culturally responsive substance use treatment are significant. Using person-first language humanizes individuals and emphasizes their intrinsic worth beyond their substance use. By acknowledging the person first, providers support a more empathetic and respectful therapeutic relationship. This form of describing someone helps remove the label of "addict" and opens the door for the individual who uses substances to understand that their substance use does not have to be who they are; it doesn't have to define them. They have an opportunity to learn about what aspects of themselves they would like to focus on that are not directly related to their substance use. Using person-first language not only reduces substance use stigma, it provides individuals a chance to see themselves beyond their addiction or substance use. This approach also fosters a sense of dignity and reduces the misconceptions often associated with substance use disorders held by society. Person-first language also recognizes the intersectionality of an individual's identity and promotes identity inclusivity. Cultural factors play a vital role in how individuals perceive themselves and their experiences with substance use. By incorporating person-first language within a culturally responsive lens, treatment providers acknowledge the influence of culture on substance use behaviors, attitudes, and recovery processes. Practicing person-first language in substance use treatment helps avoid generalizations and encourages a nuanced understanding of the individual's cultural context, ultimately leading to more effective and tailored treatment approaches.

Mental Health and Social Justice

Social justice has been more recently emphasized in the mental health profession due to several societal shifts that have occurred over the last decade. Black and Brown people being murdered by law enforcement, exacerbation of health disparities in the wake of a worldwide pandemic, political divides that have contributed to the elimination of Affirmative Action, voting rights, reduction in women's reproductive rights, and anti-trans legislation have all contributed to social justice becoming a core issue to be addressed in mental health. Unfortunately, many of the issues pertaining to social justice initiatives now are not new and have been present for several decades.

The *Encyclopedia Britannica* provides several definitions of social justice, but in defining social justice in contemporary politics, social science, and political philosophy, it states: "the fair treatment and equitable status of all individuals and social groups within a state or society. The term also is used to refer to social, political, and economic institutions, laws, or policies that collectively afford such fairness and equity and is commonly applied to movements that seek fairness, equity, inclusion, self-determination, or other goals for currently or historically oppressed, exploited, or marginalized populations."

The *Encyclopedia of Quality of Life and Well-Being Research* does not specifically define social justice, but provides common understandings of social justice by stating "Social justice is commonly viewed as a guiding principle to achieve a just society, understood both as a means as well as an end ... social justice includes a wide variety of social goals, including full and equal participation of individuals in all social institutions; fair, equitable distribution of material and nonmaterial goods (otherwise known as distributive justice); and recognition and support for the needs and rights of individuals. Social justice is also associated with a variety of processes which challenge dominance and oppression, recognize the interconnectedness and interdependence of all human beings, and champion collaboration and solidarity."

These definitions and concepts have different takes on social justice, but all generally identify the overarching concept of social justice as equity among all individuals through the ability to participate, obtain resources, and be treated fairly. As a Black woman, I wanted to be sure that I was treated fairly and seen as an individual worthy of equity in my desired profession. As such, when I got to graduate school, the graduate school that championed social justice as a core feature of the program, I was surprised when I was called a "slave driver" by a professor in one of my first graduate program classes. I was even more surprised when a cohort member asked if I ever picked cotton. I was plain dumbfounded when

I was told that only collecting data on college students of color would not be enough or empirically valid for my dissertation. Although I continued with my dissertation and was able to collect enough college students from minoritized backgrounds to determine clinical significance, feedback I received from journals regarding why my dissertation would not be published was that my sample was not diverse.

Social justice in mental health sounds nice, but practically there has been very slow progress in achieving it. The American Psychological Association has made attempts to acknowledge its part in racism and inequity through apologies and initiatives, and many other organizations are taking ownership in their part for perpetuating the inequities experienced by individuals experiencing oppression. However, there are many more opportunities to address social justice in mental health. The pervasive hold that inequities have on marginalized communities is intensified when substance use is introduced to the discussion, but like person-first language, the substance use community has simply copied the mental health profession and ignored the complexities added when considering social justice as it pertains to substance use and substance use treatment.

Substance use treatment is behind mental health treatment in the context of social justice in part because *substance use* is treated differently depending on who is using and what they are using. The crack epidemic is a prime example of inequities as they pertain to social justice, substance use, and substance use treatment. Additionally, the divergent responses between the crack epidemic and the war on drugs versus the opioid epidemic further highlight the need for social justice as it pertains to substance use and substance use treatment to be addressed. By reviewing the contrasting responses to these two crises, we can shed light on the systemic biases and social injustices that exist within substance use treatment and how it looks different from social justice in mental health treatment.

Though controversy still exists over the origins of the crack epidemic, there are several outlets that have reported that the CIA took part in assisting the onset of the crack epidemic through the purchase and distribution of crack cocaine to low-income communities of color. *Big White Lie: The CIA and the Cocaine/Crack Epidemic* was a book written by a former undercover DEA agent outlining the CIA's involvement in inequitable and illegal practices; *Freeway: Crack in the System* and *Crack: Cocaine, Corruption, & Conspiracy* are documentaries also exposing the U.S. government's active involvement in the development of and perpetuation of the crack epidemic. The response to the crack epidemic was increased and aggressive law enforcement practices, harsh criminal penalties related to crack, and disproportionate criminal penalties for powder cocaine versus crack rocks. The U.S. government named the crack epidemic as a "threat to public safety" and instituted a "War on Drugs," which continued to impose harsh penalties for individuals with addiction to crack as well as individuals who sold crack, most of whom were Black people.

The penalties for crack versus powdered cocaine were also incommensurate even though they were the same substance in different form. In 2006, the American Civil Liberties Union released a document titled *Cracks in the System: Twenty Years of the Unjust Federal Crack Cocaine Law*. This document provided grave detail about the significant penalty disparities between crack and powder cocaine, noting that the distribution of just 5 grams of crack carried a minimum 5-year federal prison sentence, while the distribution of 500 grams of powder cocaine carried the same 5-year mandatory minimum sentence. This systemic racism translated to more Black people in prison for crack distribution and fewer white people in prison for cocaine distribution. To make it plain, the amount of powder cocaine someone needed to distribute for a 5-year prison sentence was 100 times the amount of crack for the same consequence. In addition to the heavy consequences, treatment resources for crack cocaine addiction were severely lacking. Public funding for treatment was insufficient, leaving many individuals without access to adequate care. This disparity reinforced the cycle of addiction and criminalization, perpetuating social injustices.

The opioid epidemic, which emerged in the late 1990s, occurred due to overprescription of opioid medications by physicians and initially predominantly affected individuals who identified as "non-Hispanic White" (Phillips et al., 2017). The opioid epidemic was widely recognized as a public health crisis, leading to a shift in the narrative surrounding addiction. Policymakers, healthcare professionals, and the public began to view opioid addiction as a medical condition rather than a moral failing or a punishable offense, emphasizing the need for accessible treatment options. Greater attention and resources were allocated to addressing opioid addiction, resulting in increased access to evidence-based treatment modalities such as medication-assisted treatment (MAT). Efforts were made to reduce stigma and provide harm reduction strategies, aiming to prevent overdose deaths and improve outcomes for individuals affected by opioid addiction. In contrast to the crack epidemic, the response to opioid addiction was characterized by a more compassionate and public health-oriented approach.

The divergent responses to the crack and opioid epidemics highlight the underlying social injustices within substance use treatment. The crack epidemic disproportionately impacted individuals from marginalized communities, leading to punitive measures and limited access to treatment.

In contrast, the opioid epidemic, which primarily affected individuals in predominantly white communities, prompted a more compassionate and comprehensive response. These discrepancies demonstrate how uniquely systemic biases and racial inequalities influence the provision of resources, funding, and public perception of substance use disorders. Furthermore, they illustrate how mental health and substance use can look different in the context of social injustices.

Social Determinants of Health

Have you ever driven through a neighborhood and noticed the lawns? The presence of sidewalks? What about in your own neighborhood. Have you ever paid attention to the smell? Debris or lack thereof on the sidewalks? The concept of Social Determinants of Health (SDoH), according to the Office of Disease Prevention and Health Promotion, are the conditions in the environments where people are born, live, learn, work, play, worship, and age that affect a wide range of health, functioning, and quality-of-life outcomes and risks. Five domains are named based on this definition, which include economic stability, education access and quality, healthcare access and quality, neighborhood and built environment, and social and community context. Conversations around SDoH and mental wellness are vast and continuing to contribute to increased equity in mental health treatment. Additionally, the SDoH concept has gained increased focus over the last decade, as evidenced by the Office of Disease Prevention and Health Promotion committing its "Healthy People 2030's" goals specifically to addressing SDoH.

Although Social Determinants of Health are being used more often to assist the healthcare industry in understanding health and address inequities in a nuanced manner, very little focus is placed on SDoH in the context of substance use disorders. Take the questions from the beginning of this section for example. Consider you are driving through the neighborhood. Do you pay attention to the number of liquor stores you see? What about access to activities; how many parks or green spaces do you pass as you observe this neighborhood? Research has shown that liquor stores are disproportionately located in lower socioeconomic status areas with increased minoritized populations (LaVeist & Wallace Jr., 2000; Morrison et al., 2015). This was in part due to inequitable and racist land zoning practices and the denial of or disproportionate access to services for home purchasing frequently referred to as "redlining" (Egede et al., 2023). Furthermore, the lack of access to safe outdoor greenspace increases substance use risk among adolescents in "urban" identified areas (Mennis et al., 2021).

These examples of SDoH as they pertain to substance use disorders show a high need for environmental and geosocial interventions to explicitly target substance use disorders. Considering the correlation between substance use and access to safe greenspace, and the correlation between substance use and access to the substance (alcohol for example from liquor stores), provides a greater understanding to substance use treatment providers, and can be very informative for determining treatment program locations.

Parity

Engaging in belonging, justice, equity, diversity, and inclusion as it pertains to substance use treatment is another concept that is often dismissed in the mental health conversation. Parity between healthcare and mental healthcare has long been a point of contention in the healthcare industry. The concept of "Mental health is health" highlights the need to view mental health on par with physical health in terms of recognition, resources, and support within the healthcare industry. It emphasizes that mental health issues are not separate from overall health but are integral components of an individual's well-being. However, the reality is that mental health is often not given the same level of respect and importance as physical health. This disparity is more pronounced when comparing substance use treatment to physical health. Lack of parity between mental health, physical health, and substance use treatment are where the root issues are located in this conversation.

Historically, mental health services have been underfunded compared to physical healthcare services (Mahomed, 2020). The World Health Organization's Atlas Project indicated that as of 2020, the percentage of funds from government health budgets used for mental health is roughly 2%, an increase of only 1.5% since 2013. Although the percentage is not disaggregated to see what of those funds are utilized for substance use treatment, research has continued to show that substance use treatment is underfunded, leading to lack of access and increase in substance use conditions (Gibbons et al., 2023). Even with initiatives such as the Atlas Project, mental health treatment funding continues to be a significant contributor to parity issues between healthcare and mental healthcare. This disparity in resource allocation limits the availability and accessibility of mental health and substance use treatment options. Additionally, financially limited agencies attempting to provide mental health and substance use services struggle with their clients experiencing longer waiting times to receive care and limited provider availability.

Insurance coverage has also been a consistent point of reference when discussing parity between mental health, substance use, and psychical health treatments. When discussing insurance coverage, there has also historically been a clear separation of covered services for mental health treatment versus substance use treatment, with significant aspects of substance use treatment being "carved out" of insurance plans. I have a stark memory of how clinically crippling the lack of insurance coverage was when I worked in the addiction medicine department, specializing in adolescent substance use treatment at a large HMO. My client was referred to me by the child and family mental health department because, in addition to this teen's depression, she was using cannabis daily. The hospital I worked for at the time was praised for its unique ability to provide services and health insurance coverage in one place. As such, the client was able to secure a substance use intake appointment with me in the same building. My recommendation for the client was individual therapy, and a family substance use treatment program we offered at the facility. When attempting to register my client for the program, I discovered that her family's insurance had a "carve-out" for substance use programs. Though the insurance was through the hospital, it was a state-funded version of the insurance coverage, and with that version, substance use treatment could only be obtained at a facility that accepted state-funded insurance. This client was able to receive all her care through the hospital except substance use treatment. This example provides several issues that exist regarding equitable substance use treatment and the lack of parity between mental health and substance use treatment from an institutionalized standpoint. The client's family was able to retain insurance coverage, which is a known financial barrier to begin with, however, the insurance coverage secured by the family only allowed for physical health treatment and mental health treatment, leaving substance use treatment to be obtained by a different agency. Barriers to entry, like this one, are one of many reasons people seeking substance use treatment, especially individuals from minoritized backgrounds, end up falling through the cracks.

The separation of insurance coverage regarding mental health treatment services and substance use treatment services also increases stigma of substance use conditions. It is well established that the stigma regarding substance use conditions contributes to the disparity in treatment funding, access, and respect. Insurance companies reinforce this stigma by not funding, or underfunding, needed substance use treatment interventions. In essence, insurance companies are indirectly saying "if you have a broken leg, we will cover your treatment. If you have depression, we will only cover your treatment if it significantly impairs other aspects of your life to the point of low or no functioning, but if you have an addiction, you are on your own."

An additional barrier to equitable treatment of substance use and treatment parity among physical and mental health is lack of integration of treatment. The separation between physical healthcare and mental healthcare, and furthermore, substance use treatment perpetuates a fragmented approach to healthcare delivery. Consider this example. An individual is in a car accident and goes to the hospital for injuries to be assessed. At the hospital, the individual can get an x-ray completed, vitals taken, and a thorough physical assessment to identify any other potential injuries that need to be addressed. All of this occurs in one place, making it easy for the individual to receive immediate care for what was discovered as a broken leg from the car accident. Additionally, all these procedures and assessments are covered by the person's insurance, so they can receive care to address their injuries without having to pay. What is not assessed is the individual's mental health after experiencing a traumatic event. The car accident left another individual unconscious and the individual in this example saw the other person before being taken to the emergency room. The doctor treating the individual happens to have a background in mental health, and as a result, makes a referral to the psychiatry department for this individual to receive a psychological intake. However, the process for the individual to obtain an intake is arduous, takes more time, and does not occur in the same building or same day as the other physical assessments.

Using this same example, if the individual arrived at the hospital and tests revealed that the person was intoxicated, instead of treatment referral, the police would be contacted, and the individual could be arrested for driving under the influence. At no point would substance use treatment be discussed in conjunction with, or in addition to the potential criminal consequences. By treating mental health as a distinct and separate entity, opportunities for holistic and integrated care are missed. By treating substance use as a crime first, stigma and discrimination are perpetuated at the system level and person-centered care is not implemented.

Many physical health conditions have mental health components, and conversely, mental health conditions can have physical manifestations. The same concept goes for substance use conditions as they pertain to physical and mental health conditions. The Mental Health Parity and Addiction Equity Act of 2008 attempted to address the limitations set by insurance companies regarding access to mental health and substance use treatment by removing insurance company's ability to impose annual or lifetime dollar limits on mental health benefits that were not equitable compared to limits placed on medical benefits. However, there is still a deficit in the implementation and effectiveness of the law. This lack of progress prompted the need for new initiatives and federal regulations to be implemented to help reduce the disparity in treatment access and funding. Some examples include the elimination of the X waiver through the Biden administration, which was a certification required for clinicians to prescribe medication for opioid addiction, and the World Health Organization's Atlas Project, which provides target goals and data related to how well a country is implementing changes to achieve parity in mental health treatment. Though these initiatives are helpful, there are still significant changes that need to occur with policy, health insurance coverage, and overall conceptualization of substance use conditions to achieve parity.

Intersectionality of Mental Health and Substance Use

Up to this point, this book has shown several reasons why understanding substance use treatment and providing culturally responsive substance use treatment specifically, are critical to the quality-of-care individuals who have substance use conditions receive. Additionally, historical accounts of how substance use has been thought of separately from mental health treatment has been emphasized. One might think intersectionality of mental health and substance use appears counter to the reason for the book, and negates all points made prior to this section. However, understanding intersectionality of mental health and substance use is actually one of the key reasons this book is so important. The concept of intersectionality as defined by the Center for Intersectional Justice is the "way in which systems of inequality based on gender, race, ethnicity, sexual orientation, gender identity, disability, class, and other forms of discrimination "intersect" to create unique dynamics and effects." Merriam-Webster defines intersectionality as "the complex, cumulative way in which the effects of multiple forms of discrimination (such as racism, sexism, and classism) combine, overlap, or intersect especially in the experiences of marginalized individuals or groups." Considering the intersectionality of mental health and substance use to provide culturally responsive substance use treatment means looking at cultural and systemic barriers that contribute to substance use conditions and mental health conditions. Taking these complex aspects of an individual into consideration when conceptualizing their condition and developing treatment interventions is a key component in making the treatment culturally responsive.

What has been discussed is the issue of absorbing substance use treatment in mental health treatment. This means not taking into consideration the systemic and institutionalized practices that may lead someone to substance use or cause a marginalized individual to be misdiagnosed or underdiagnosed. To effectively provide culturally responsive substance use treatment, awareness of and acknowledgment of systemic injustices, oppression, and institutionalized racism need to occur. All aspects of an individual's life experiences have a profound impact on their mental health and their own understanding of their substance use.

The Grammy- and Emmy-award-winning and Academy- and Golden-Globe-nominated artist Kendrick Lamar is impeccable at utilizing his art to paint verbal pictures of his experience beautifully and authentically as a Black man who is working through generational curses and historical trauma. He uses his music to share his experience with the world, and in doing this, he gives words to those who share his experiences but struggle to articulate them. In one song, "Mother I Sober," his lyrics paint a picture of dealing with an experience of seeing his mother be physically abused when he was 5 years old, feeling guilt for not "doing" anything, historical trauma of slavery, rape, and sexism:

> Mother's brother said he got revenge for my mother's face
> Black and blue, the image of my queen that I can't erase
> 'Til this day can't look her in the eyes, pain is taking over
> Blame myself, you never felt guilt 'til you felt it sober

In this example, Kendrick describes how he views his mother, as a queen, the image of her face after being beat, and the pain he experiences when he looks at her. He also states that he blames himself for this and alludes to drowning the guilt of this pain with substance use, which had kept him from experiencing the pain and guilt. He ends the verse stating that he now actually feels guilt because he is sober. The intersectionality of mental health and substance use is illustrated through this song in that the substance use is more than a coping strategy for several traumatic experiences that have occurred. Taking the way intersectionality is defined, the overlap of childhood trauma, lack of safety and trust in the establishment due to generational violence (as described in other parts of the song), post-traumatic slave syndrome, prejudices, and discrimination all contribute to one's engagement in substances. Using this framework to better understand one's substance use will assist in better understanding culturally responsive ways to address the substance use. Truthfully, it is less about the substance use and more about the systemic oppression, institutionalized racism, generational trauma, and inequitable access to affirming treatment that need to be addressed. Validation of the role these issues play in an individual's substance use help develop comprehensive treatment.

Overall, considering the intersectionality of mental health and substance use will improve the way providers and organizations conduct treatment for individuals of marginalized communities. Additionally, addressing how the organization or provider may inadvertently contribute to these injustices and making changes accordingly increases the level of safety individuals from marginalized communities feel if and when they do seek treatment.

References

Baker, E. A., Hamilton, M., Culpepper, D., McCune, G., & Silone, G. (2022). The effect of person-first language on attitudes toward people with addiction. *Journal of Addictions & Offender Counseling*, *43*(1), 38–49. 10.1002/jaoc.12102

Cohen, I. G., & Mello, M. M. (2020). Big data, big tech, and protecting patient privacy. *NEJM Catalyst Innovations in Care Delivery*, *1*(6). 10.1056/CAT.20.0414

Disrupting stigma: How understanding, empathy, and connection can improve outcomes for families affected by substance use and mental disorders. *National Center on Substance Abuse and Child Welfare*.

Dunn, D. S., & Andrews, E. E. (2015). Person-first and identity-first language: Developing psychologists' cultural competence using disability language. *American Psychologist*, *70*(3), 255–264. 10.1037/a0038636

Egede, L. E., Walker, R. J., Campbell, J. A., Linde, S., Hawks, L. C., & Burgess, K. M. (2023). Modern day consequences of historic redlining: Finding a path forward. *Journal of General Internal Medicine*, *38*(6), 1534–1537. 10.1007/s11606-023-08051-4

FiveThirtyEight. (February 9, 2022). Redlining in America. https://projects.fivethirtyeight.com/redlining/

Gibbons, J., Harris, S., Solomon, K., Sugarman, O., Hardy, C., Saloner, B., (2023). Increasing overdose deaths among Black Americans: A review of the literature. *The Lancet Psychiatry*. 10.1016/S2215-0366(23)00119-0

Johns Hopkins Bloomberg School of Public Health. (2014, September 23). Study: Public feels more negative toward people with drug addiction than those with mental illness. https://publichealth.jhu.edu/2014/study-public-feels-more-negative-toward-people-with-drug-addiction-than-those-with-mental-illness

LaVeist, T. A., & Wallace, J. M., Jr. (2000). Health risk and inequitable distribution of liquor stores in African American neighborhood. *Social Science & Medicine (1982)*, *51*(4), 613–617. 10.1016/s0277-9536(00)00004-6

Mahomed, F. (2020). Addressing the problem of severe underinvestment in mental health and well-being from a human rights perspective. *Health and Human Rights*, *22*(1), 35–49.

Mennis, J., Li, X., Meenar, M., Coatsworth, J. D., McKeon, T. P., & Mason, M. J. (2021). Residential greenspace and urban adolescent substance use: Exploring interactive effects with peer network health, sex, and executive function. *International Journal of Environmental Research and Public Health*, *18*(4), 1611. 10.3390/ijerph18041611

Mennis, J., Stahler, G. J., & Mason, M. J. (2016). Risky substance use environments and addiction: A new frontier for environmental justice research. *International Journal of Environmental Research and Public Health*, *13*(6), 607. 10.3390/ijerph13060607

Morrison, C., Gruenewald, P. J., & Ponicki, W. R. (2015). Socioeconomic determinants of exposure to alcohol outlets. *Journal of Studies on Alcohol and Drugs*, *76*(3), 439–446. 10.15288/jsad.2015.76.439

National Academies of Sciences, Engineering, and Medicine; Health and Medicine Division; Board on Health Sciences Policy; Committee on Pain Management and Regulatory Strategies to Address Prescription Opioid Abuse; Phillips, J. K., Ford, M. A., & Bonnie, R. J. (Eds.). (2017 Jul 13). *Pain Management and the Opioid Epidemic: Balancing Societal and Individual Benefits and Risks of Prescription Opioid Use*. Washington (DC): National Academies Press (US). 4, Trends in Opioid Use, Harms, and Treatment. Available from: https://www.ncbi.nlm.nih.gov/books/NBK458661/

U.S. Department of Health and Human Services. (n.d.). Social Determinants of Health. *Healthy People 2030*. https://health.gov/healthypeople/priority-areas/social-determinants-health

Urban Institute. (March 15, 2023). Ghosts of Housing Discrimination Reach Beyond Redlining. https://www.urban.org/features/ghosts-housing-discrimination-reach-beyond-redlining

Yang, L. H., Wong, L. Y., Grivel, M. M., & Hasin, D. S. (2017). Stigma and substance use disorders: An international phenomenon. *Current Opinion in Psychiatry*, *30*(5), 378–388. 10.1097/YCO.0000000000000351

Culturally Responsive Substance Use Treatment

What It REALLY Means

As outlined in previous chapters, substance use treatment has a long history of being an unfortunate afterthought in healthcare treatment. Initially labeled a "moral issue," the way we understood addiction removed any possibility that substance use could be treatable. Disparaging social depictions of substance use and the disproportionate impact that substances had on minoritized communities was harmful and contributed to significant aspects of institutionalized racism. This continues to be illustrated through punishment instead of treatment for minoritized individuals experiencing substance use challenges. The ups and downs of substance use are also depicted through prescription medications. The story arc of prescription medications is, "we found a miracle drug! Prescribe it to everyone, for everything, all the time! It solves all the problems!" to "oops! Turns out this is highly addictive. Sorry, this one creates worse symptoms. Take it off the shelves and ban it worldwide!" The medical profession is often prematurely excited about prescription medications that show promise to "cure" mental health conditions, and what we have seen through history is those medications often end up LEADING to addiction. Once this happens, a person becomes labeled as an "addict" or "pill popper" and the misuse of prescription medications grows exponentially.

The Culturally Responsive Substance use Treatment (CRST pronounced "Crust") Framework considers all aspects of a person (Lived Identities) and the intersectionality of those lived identities with their Life Stage, Recovery Lifestyle, and various aspects of society (Systemic Impact), to inform a culturally responsive, comprehensive, and flexible treatment approach. I define cultural responsiveness more broadly as "the conscious act of responding to the cultural needs of others as defined by them." The CRST Framework is rooted in this definition of cultural responsiveness. There are aspects of the framework that are informed by systems and societal impact, however, the core of the framework, as

DOI: 10.4324/9781032708829-7

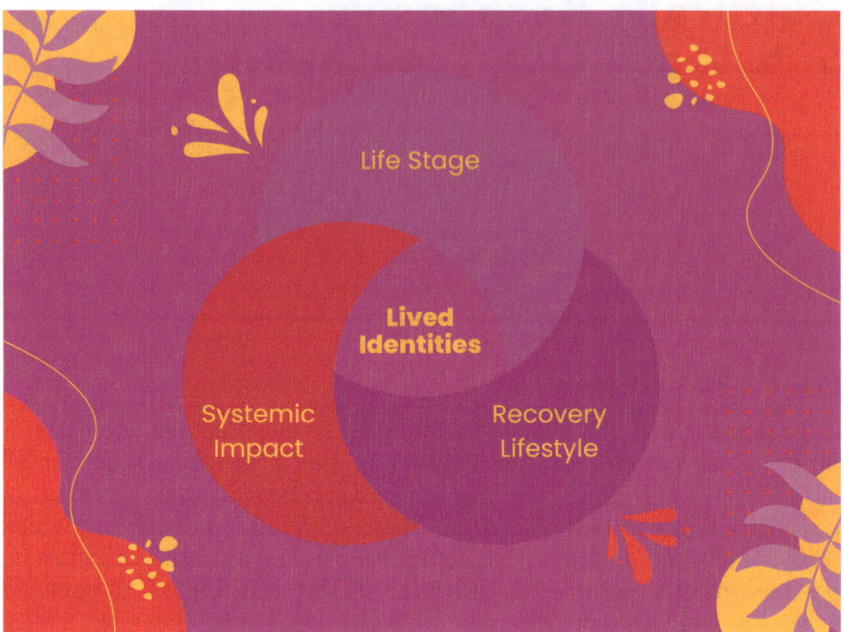

Figure 7.1 Culturally Responsive Substance Use Treatment (CRST) Framework.

exemplified by being in the center, are the Lived Identities as they are reported and experienced by the individual. This core is what influences and is influenced by Life Stage, Recovery Lifestyle, and Systemic Impact (Figure 7.1).

Theoretical underpinnings of the CRST Framework come from Dr. Janet Helms' Identity Development Theories (Helms, 1990) and Dr. Nancy Boyd-Franklin's Multisystems approach to the treatment of Black families (Boyd-Franklin, 1989). These models have not only been tremendously influential in the profession of psychology, but both scholars, Black women identified, have revolutionized treatment practices at the individual, group, and system level by restructuring our conceptualization of identity for the betterment of humanity. The CRST framework is intended to continue the advancement of the work done by Dr. Helms and Dr. Boyd-Franklin.

The CRST framework seeks to empower historically minoritized and marginalized individuals to share their Lived Identities that are most salient to their Life Stage, Recovery Lifestyle, and Systemic Impact. The concept of Lived Identities does not remove the culturally oppressive experiences individuals encounter, which is typically a byproduct of traditional substance use treatment, instead, it allows individuals to name the experiences themselves as they relate to their identities. The intention behind centering the framework around one's multiple Lived Identities is to help expand that person's perception of their identity to be more encompassing of the multiple identities they carry. Additionally, this allows individuals to bring more of themselves to treatment and provides clinicians with a more comprehensive and integrated understanding of the person. This framework also highlights the interplay between the portions, as they all influence each other.

Lived Identities

The Lived Identities portion of the CRST framework is best described as the "active ingredient" for the rest of the framework. Lived Identities alone can bring up a wide array of topics, discussions, and disagreements, but do not provide much direction. Lived Identities in the context of culturally responsive substance use treatment present a rich opportunity for providers, organizations, and systems to become more culturally informed and aware regarding their treatment practices. One's Lived Identities refers to the identities an individual possesses and their lived experiences that come because of those identities. Additionally, these Lived Identities are important to the individual and the lived experiences have had an impact on their life in some way. Lived Identities goes beyond one's demographics by pairing lived experiences with salient identities that an individual distinguishes as important to them because of those lived experiences.

The concept of Lived Identities is critical to culturally responsive substance use treatment. Current models of substance use treatment blatantly ignore one's Lived Identities and overemphasize the substance use or addiction. Core models of treatment for substance use are rooted in stigmatizing language instead of person-first language. These existing treatment approaches are contributing to the inability for the profession to move past stigma and into equitable treatment. Removing an individual's identities or limiting their identity to being an "addict" not only dehumanizes the individual, but it is counter to minoritized and marginalized individual mental wellness overall. Individuals from minoritized and marginalized communities are historically reduced to their race or ethnicity in society; substance use treatment in its current state does the same thing. Just because anyone can develop a substance use condition doesn't mean we can assume people who develop a substance use condition are all the same. Sports are an example of how mutual respect, not sameness, is what builds community. People who play soccer have that in common. They all enjoy the game and are on the same team. However, the team is made up of individuals from varying backgrounds, have different lived experiences that led them to soccer, and have different perspectives about the game. The uniting component is that they are on the same team and share a love for the sport. Their different perspectives, identities, and experiences are what make for a strong team because their differences are respected and appreciated. This is how substance use treatment needs to look. The commonality may be the substance use condition, but the unique identities and lived experiences are different and should be respected as such.

Having a substance use condition can provide opportunity for commonality and community, but it should not be at the expense of an individual's other Lived Identities. Part of culturally responsive substance use treatment is assisting the individual in finding their identities outside of their substance use. Another aspect of focusing on identities is to validate the experiences of minoritized and marginalized individuals. Validation can have profound benefit to building trust among communities of color who have historically been mistreated in healthcare systems.

An example of this would be an individual who identifies as a queer Black father. This person expresses these three terms as principal identities. They have lived experiences as Queer, Black, and Father, respectively. Notice this individual chose the term "Father" rather than "Parent," although they also identify as "Queer." This is because the lived experience of a "Black Parent" is different from the lived experience of a "Black Father," which is also different from the lived experience of a "Queer Parent." These Lived Identities may not be the only ones experienced by this individual. As treatment progresses, these Lived Identities may become less leading, or they may shift over time. The key is to prioritize learning, developing an understanding for one's Lived Identities as the primary approach.

In the CRST Framework as a provider, making and maintaining a "clinical space" for clients to explore their Lived Identities is part of the initial rapport building process. Initial sessions should begin with curiosity about how an individual describes themselves or what identities are most present for the client in the moment. To accomplish this, the following questions can be utilized:

"Can you share what identities you most align with in this moment?"

"What would you say are the most important parts of your identity for you?"

"I want to review the demographic information you provided with you so I am better able to understand which identities are most salient for you currently. Is that OK with you, or would you rather tell me without us reviewing the form together?"

Note that all prompts and examples need to be followed up with a request for elaboration from the client. A simple "can you tell me what makes them important for you" can provide your client with "clinical space" to share. This approach not only has the potential to help build rapport, but it validates the client and their lived experience. Validation is an extremely effective tool for substance use treatment. In providing this clinical space, you are also showing to the client that you see them for more than their substance use, and you are developing a solid foundation for recovery work. The CRST Framework is not limited to individual providers. In organizational settings, expanding demographic question data will provide more context regarding Lived Identities for the clients served which can inform more appropriate and culturally responsive program development and meaningful policy change. Using the CRST Framework, this can be achieved through equitable data management strategies. Diversifying the type of data collected to include Social Determinants of Health (SDoH) paints a more accurate picture of the collective group "identities" being served by your organization, which allows you to more effectively target the issues present in your community. Additionally, disaggregating your data to be more reflective of intergroup identities provides more accurate information to your staff delivering services and enhances their ability to provide more equitable and culturally responsive substance use treatment. Finally, diversifying the way you collect data (ex: utilization of transcription tools during the end of an appointment instead of mailing surveys), increases your response rate and yields richer content to be used for service improvement systemwide. Lived Identities are not limited to the three that will be covered in this section. Race, gender identity/sexual orientation, and neurodiversity are emphasized because these Lived Identities are highly correlated with substance use and co-occurring disorders. Additional considerations for other diverse identities will be addressed at the end of the book.

Racial Identity Development

Dr. Helms's Identity Development Models posit that identity development includes recognizing that identity is developed through an individual's context in various social groups, their lived experiences based on their perceived identities, and varying forms of oppression. As a result, healthy identity development involves accepting all parts of self, while appreciating the uniqueness and differences of others (Adames et al., 2023). These concepts are embedded in the CRST Framework. Race as a social construct will be discussed more as a component of the CRST framework in the Systemic Impact section. Allowing individuals to share and explore their Lived Identities promotes integration of their various identities and provides an opportunity to develop an appreciation for themselves holistically. In doing this, individuals are also able to develop an appreciation for the diversity and uniqueness of others. It is imperative to note that an individual's Lived Identities are what THEY identify as their Lived Identities. This is not an invitation for providers to place assumptions on individuals or suggest identities to an individual based on an individual's external presentation. Helms's Racial Identity Social Interaction Model (Helms & Cook, 1999) surfaces how social interactions and social power (ex: provider-patient) influence racial identity. This concept, as well as making assumptions will be addressed in the System Impact section of this chapter. The key component for the CRST Framework is that racial identity is essential to the process of culturally responsive treatment. There is an inherent power differential in therapeutic relationships. As such, in the CRST Framework, providers are responsible not only for exploring and understanding their own racial identity development, but they are also responsible for remaining aware of their own racial identity as it pertains to their client in treatment.

Even if there is a shared phenotype between provider and client, opening the door for discussion is an important component of the Lived Identities portion of the CRST Framework. Emphasis is placed on the "Lived" part of Lived Identities when providers have similar identities to their client because the lived experiences may be different and making assumptions that are incorrect have the potential to destroy the therapeutic relationship before it is developed. This is also why the CRST Framework heavily emphasizes providers identify their own stage of racial identity development as a part of providing culturally responsive substance use treatment. The CRST Framework emphasizes the work to be done at the organizational level as it pertains to identity development in the context of race as well. Adames et al. (2023) showcase the expansion of the Helms Racial Identity Social Interaction Model for organizations, outlining four organizational racial identity schemas that explain organizational identity stages. For the CRST Framework, organizations are encouraged to work toward that of Integrative Awareness. In practice, this looks like shifting policy and engaging in proper training to promote cultural responsiveness in substance use treatment among staff. It also looks like integrating more culturally responsive practices within the organization. See Chapter 3 for more examples of what Integrative Awareness can look like at the system level as it pertains to culturally responsive substance use treatment.

Gender Identity and Sexual Orientation

Individuals with Lived Identities that include gender identity and sexual orientation have been aggressively marginalized in substance use treatment.

People seeking residential treatment have been placed in hostile housing environments where they are emotionally, verbally, and sometimes physically abused. These individuals have expressed in various treatment settings the discomfort with being placed in a gender-specific group due to their physical appearance and have even engaged in "treatment noncompliance" by skipping program requirements that force them to deny parts of themselves for the sake of treatment. Individuals with Lived Identities that include a diverse sexual orientation must consider if someone in treatment is "uncomfortable" with someone of a different sexual orientation, which adds to their mental load of seeking recovery themselves. The risk of being "outed" before someone is comfortable sharing their sexual orientation is also a factor in the inequitable substance use treatment practices we see currently. All these examples are abhorrent and antithetical to culturally responsive substance use treatment, and yet, they occur constantly. These incidents contribute to individuals with Lived Identities related to gender identity and sexual orientation not being their full selves in treatment and contribute to these individuals leaving treatment prematurely or avoiding treatment altogether.

The CRST Framework aims to bring the issues that people with these Lived Identities to the front of treatment. In doing so, the framework promotes awareness of the problems individuals with these Lived Identities face and places the provider in the role of addressing these concerns before they happen. As mentioned, the Lived Identities portion of the CRST Framework encourages discussion of Lived Identities in the beginning of treatment. As it pertains to gender identity and sexual orientation, discussing these Lived Identities in the initial stages of treatment gives the provider insight into potential barriers to treatment. The provider's role here is to prioritize client safety. Inquiring about any negative past treatment experiences related to the individual's gender identity or sexual orientation provides insight regarding what the provider needs to keep in mind and protect the client from. This may look like starting groups with guidelines pertaining to the use of chosen names or making clear statements about group members not making assumptions about other group members. At the system level, this looks like developing policy that offers accommodations for individuals with these Lived Identities. Some policy examples are having different living arrangements for nonbinary individuals, immediate consequences for individuals who engage in homophobic behavior in any way or using first initials instead of names as part of your program guidelines. Implementing these institutional changes reflect to individuals with Lived Identities pertaining to gender identity and sexual orientation that they are safe, and the organization sees them as a whole person. It is also important to note that obtaining consultation for your specific organization based on demographic and geographic information will help to develop a robust and equitable culturally responsive substance use treatment program for your system.

Neurodiversity

What some would call an "invisible identity," individuals with neurodiverse Lived Identities have experiences that are anything but invisible. Furthermore, substance use treatment programs and approaches are so myopic that sometimes I wonder how any program can boast cultural responsiveness. Treatment programs were not built, nor are they maintained for individuals with neurodiverse Lived Identities. The benefit of having Lived Identities at the core of the CRST Framework is that as a provider, you will discover early on if your client has neurodiverse Lived Identities. This knowledge presents providers with useful information to develop a culturally responsive treatment plan. Although it is helpful for providers, individuals with Lived Identities pertaining to neurodiversity offer substantial benefit to organizations and systems by promoting the development of more robust and comprehensive treatment programs.

The CRST Framework centers on how systems and organizations need to change regarding individuals with neurodiverse Lived Identities. Most programs offer individual therapy, group therapy, and case management services. This is outdated and limited to individuals without Lived Identities of neurodiversity. Programs instead need to structure themselves to incorporate technology as it evolves. This might look like VR activities as a group. Instead of sitting and talking, incorporating nature as a component of treatment by giving cohorts of individuals garden beds to tend to as part of their treatment program. These adjustments do not just benefit individuals with Neurodiverse Lived Identities, they benefit everyone in treatment. At the provider level, the goal is to develop a space where your client can communicate in the way that is best for them. This may look like using a card game or board to ask questions during the session. This may look like having access to art supplies during initial sessions to allow the client to draw while engaging in treatment. It may look as simple as sitting on the floor where there is more tactile diversity during sessions. Regardless of what it looks like, using the definition of culturally responsive substance use treatment, respond to the needs of the client, as defined by the client.

Life Stage

The CRST framework is intersectional by design, however, Life Stage is located at the top of the framework intentionally. Life Stage impacts Lived Identities simply because the longer you live, the more Lived Identities you develop. An individual's Lived Identities and Recovery Lifestyle shift the most based on their Life Stage. Similarly, the longer you live, the more opportunities there are for Systemic Impact Experiences. An individual's Life Stage can also have profound impacts on the other portions of the framework. The overall concept of Life Stage in the CRST framework is that it allows the provider to consider what is important to the client based on their Life Stage. Through the framework, what is important to the client informs the providers of intervention strategies. However, what matters to clients differs as their Life Stage shifts. Additionally, Life Stages come with their own cultural underpinnings, which is why Life Stage is an important part of culturally responsive substance use treatment. Current treatment models are severely lacking when it comes to adolescent substance use treatment and older adult substance use treatment. Most existing treatment approaches are only marginally "adapted" for different Life Stages. The CRST framework was developed in part to fill the large gap that exists in culturally responsive treatment for individuals in different Life Stages.

Youth

Working in juvenile corrections, I was able to see the pain experienced in the youth Life Stage very intimately. The typical developmental stage of adolescence is already remarkably difficult, but being incarcerated in addition to that was another level of difficulty. As adults, we often forget about how hard this Life Stage really is. Our bodies are changing, our feelings are complex, and our identities are transitioning from being informed by core family values to being informed by social ones. Our familial relationships are often strained during this Life Stage, making substance use treatment more challenging, and we are attempting to seek independence while still not being fully prepared to go out on our own.

The youth Life Stage also presents the unique challenge of having some Lived Identities while not feeling confident in any identities. This Life Stage is packed with confusion and adding substance use treatment often breeds resentment. To prevent making this Life Stage any more difficult than it already is, the CRST framework focuses on reducing confusion and assisting the client in defining what identity means to them. This involves understanding the client's existing Lived Identities from the client as well as their family. Since this Life Stage is full of developmental shifts, having family involvement in treatment is critical. Family involvement, however, is defined uniquely within the CRST framework and is also informed by the multisystems approach. Family, as it is described within the CRST framework extends to chosen family, teachers, mentors, spiritual leaders, neighbors, and family friends. The important point is that the young individual you are working with has the autonomy to identify a safe or trusted adult in their life who can participate in their treatment. Removing the systemic barrier placed in treatment of adult involvement in treatment having to be a parent is what makes the CRST framework culturally responsive. Involvement from a trusted or safe adult in treatment may look like phone consultations between the adult and the provider that is also shared with the adolescent.

If parents are involved in treatment, it is important to create a safe space between the client and their parent. This looks like creating therapeutic expectations, talking to the youth about how to approach difficult topics before bringing in parents, and being clear and direct about your role and limitations with the family up front. Youth can smell a fake miles away, so ensuring that you are authentic will go a long way. Additionally, having parent involvement is beneficial if possible, but treatment should not be limited to parent involvement. Regardless of parent involvement, the adolescent needs to be able to identify other safe or trusted adults that can be involved in treatment. In many cultures, there is a saying that "it takes a village to raise a child" and the same concept is promoted in the CRST framework. The more trusted adults involved in treatment, the more positively impacted this Life Stage becomes.

Emerging Adults

The term emerging adults describes individuals between the ages of 18 and 29 and is often referred to as "the in-between" age due to the Life Stage experienced during this age. Emerging adults are old enough to engage in most, if not all "adult" activities. Gambling, legal drinking and smoking, and voting are all privileges that are bestowed upon individuals in the emerging adult life stage. Additionally, this is the Life Stage where individuals begin to explore different identities through academic endeavors, career development, and intimate partnerships. As such, this Life Stage comes with its own unique cultural shifts that need to be considered from the CRST framework. Seeing as this Life Stage is packed with new opportunities, it is important to encourage and promote the exploration of identities. In the CRST framework, the provider focuses on helping the client discover what types of experiences they want to live and what types of identities they want to have. Addressing identities at this Life Stage are critical because as they become crystalized, if an individual returns to use, they will have these solidified identities to return to as part of their treatment.

This Life Stage also presents opportunities for providers to promote healthy lifestyle practices that can become a normal and consistent part of the emerging adult's life. When utilizing the CRST framework for treatment at this Life Stage, it is also important to consider family involvement from the perspective of the client. Typical substance use treatment practices are heavily oriented in Western individualized culture, and this is not conducive to many minoritized and marginalized individuals. Community and family still play a major role in the lives of emerging adults from diverse backgrounds and provide valuable context regarding the existing Lived Identities of the emerging adult. Encouraging independence can be counterproductive to culturally responsive treatment and can hinder providers from seeing the whole "picture" of the emerging adult.

Consider a client who is drinking heavily and is in college. He does not have a history of significant drinking behavior but continues to be referred for therapy due to his drinking behavior. You inquire about his family substance use history and there is no evidence of substance use concerns among family members. The client informs you that he "doesn't know" why he is drinking so much but has insight regarding some anxiety he reported. He shares that he had anxiety in high school but managed it well and without medication. You attempt to provide him with harm reduction strategies like drinking a cup of water in between alcohol beverages and he is still unable to control his drinking. It seems like nothing is working because he clearly cannot remain sober, he isn't able to restrict his use, and he does not want to take medication.

Utilizing the CRST framework in this case example, based on his Life Stage your efforts are geared toward helping the client identify the experiences he wants to live and the identities he wants to have. You also want to understand his community. In the CRST framework you would first inquire about the experiences he wants to live by asking something like, "you are drinking a lot and it seems troubling to you, what type of life experiences do you want to have here?" Your client shares that he wants to connect with people, but he is having difficulty. This is where considerations of his Lived Identities become important. A client in the emerging adult Life Stage generally is looking for their shared identity group. If your client is not connecting with people, he likely struggled with his Lived Identities in his youth. With this, you ask, "what type of people do you want to connect with?" Your client shares that he is unsure and that he just misses home. He becomes closed off and it is now challenging to continue building rapport. In the CRST framework, this is a good opportunity to develop an understanding of your patient's community as well as what his Lived Identities may have been prior to college. You enquire about where his family lives and you discover that they are about 4 hours away from the client. Because of the distance he shares he is not able to see them much. You ask if the client would be comfortable with you talking to his family, not about his alcohol use but about ways to increase visits. Your client agrees for you to talk to his mother and signs a consent form.

Per his mother, your client went to a predominately White high school and was often treated inequitably due to his Mexican American identity. She mentioned that he was a bit anxious, but it was managed well because he had family members who all lived close by, and he did not spend much time with school friends outside of his family and his friends from church. He was well-liked, but his biggest challenge was being one of the only Mexican Americans in his class.

With this insight, from the CRST framework, you now know that one of your client's Lived Identities is Mexican American. You may have had that information from the demographic intake form, but since the client has not discussed this explicitly in treatment, you had not inquired about it. The CRST framework prompts providers to begin treatment with the exploration of client Lived Identities. It is not the responsibility of minoritized and marginalized clients to initiate topics that are uncomfortable, such as race or gender identity. It is the provider's responsibility to make space for clients to share Lived Identities that are most important to them. One Lived Identity of this client is Mexican American. He is close with his family, and this is his first experience not having familial support close by. This college is likely triggering his anxiety about his Lived Identity because it is also predominately White. As the provider, taking this Life Stage into consideration, helping the client identify what identities he would like to have is the focus. To do this, you **share** what information you gleaned from the client's mother regarding his Lived Identity and **inquire** about his experiences in high school. As the provider, you also want to inquire about aspects of his Lived Identity that he enjoyed and would like to expand on in college. In learning about his Lived Identity as a Mexican American, you **validate** the minoritized experiences he shares with you.

Your client shares his desire to maintain his Mexican American Lived Identity and together, you identify that his excessive drinking behaviors are a result of his lack of connection to this Lived Identity. In this Life Stage, one of the biggest challenges emerging adults face is their lack of awareness of resources available to them. In the youth Life Stage, individuals are still receiving assistance in navigating life and the world. In this Life Stage, the provider also serves as a **resource guide** for the client. The important and distinguishing factor for providing resources to clients in this Life Stage is to ask if specific resources would be helpful before providing them. In this case example, that would look like the provider making a statement like, "As we explore your Lived Identity as a Mexican American, and knowing this is an Identity important to you, would it be helpful for you to have resources related to LatinX organizations on campus?" In many cases, providers will jump ahead and pull resources together to give to clients without considering if they would be helpful. Taking the CRST approach to asking about resources before providing them gives clients at this Life Stage an opportunity to adequately articulate their needs with your support.

The emerging adult Life Stage is much more focused on exploring and developing more Lived Identities. The provider's role at this Life Stage is to provide space for individuals to share their Lived Identities, inquire about Lived Identities individuals would like to carry into this Life Stage, validate the minoritized and marginalized experiences had by the individual, and provide resources based on the client's Lived Identity goals.

Adults

In the adult Life Stage, individuals have generally become comfortable with their Lived Identities, but new experiences and the need to "plan" for the future become more important. This Life Stage can also be overwhelming for individuals, but for different reasons. Solidified intimate partnerships and careers are leading this Life Stage. Additionally, this Life Stage is often where the Lived Identities of parenthood and caregiver for aging parents become prominent. The combination of these established Lived Identities and these new Lived Identities can cause immense pressure and stress in this Life Stage. These stressful Life Stage transitions and solidified Lived Identities often contribute to substance use. Because of this, The CRST framework in this Life Stage has the provider focus on understanding the source of the pressure/stress and promoting the individual giving themselves grace in this Life Stage. Giving grace means acknowledging the difficulties an individual is experiencing within the context of their Lived Identities; recognizing the challenges and giving oneself permission to take breaks, be human, and overall, be kind to oneself.

In the next illustration of how the CRST framework looks at this Life Stage, you are working with a high-achieving individual who has developed unhealthy prescription substance use. He is seeking treatment because he is concerned about his family life. This individual has established Lived Identities that include the following: first-generation college graduate, born of parents who migrated from Nigeria, and engineer. His new Lived Identities include Husband, Black Father, and care-support for his aging parents. You have this information because you spent initial treatment sessions exploring what the client identified as his primary Lived Identities. The client shared with you that his career is successful and he is proud of his established Lived Identities, but he feels very stressed out at work, and unsure of his new Lived Identities because he has never done them before. He also shares with you that his Lived Identity as a Nigerian man involves being strong and "keeping it together." He tells you therapy is not something he is totally comfortable with yet.

You will notice that there has not yet been an explicit discussion about his substance use. Providers have an ethical responsibility to understand an individual's substance use, but to *address* the substance use from a culturally responsive framework, understanding the whole person is critical. Your client shares that he uses prescription medications to keep him alert at work and to help him stay awake with his child so that his partner can get rest. He also shares that he goes to his parent's home every other day after work to bring groceries and check in on them. His father recently had a fall and is not allowed to drive, so when your client visits his parents, he takes his mother on her errands as well. As mentioned, the CRST framework in this Life Stage prioritizes understanding the stress and pressure experienced by the client. In this example, validating that your client is attempting to achieve perfection in all his Lived Identities is important. You have learned from your client that this way of life is not abnormal for him given his Nigerian Lived Identity, so instead of attempting to reduce the amount of work that is likely contributing to his stress and his prescription substance use, your role as the provider is to help your client understand the objective difficulties associated with his new Lived Identities as Black Father, Husband, ad care-support for aging parents. Understanding where the client feels like he is "failing" and facilitating the use of neutral language, as well as providing perspective for the client will promote the client giving himself grace with his new Lived Identities.

Some specific ways to assist clients in giving themselves grace in this Life Stage using the CRST framework are to:

- Facilitate exploration of what the established Lived Identities will look like once the client has had time to get adjusted to them
- Explore the client's established Lived Identities and assist the client in remembering what those Lived Identities looked like when they were new. (Consider helping the client explore their Lived Identities from their youth and emerging adult Life Stages).
- Seek input from client about natural and nonmedicated ways to reduce stress encouraging activities and behaviors that are realistic and in alignment with their Recovery Lifestyle

An example of the third point with the same client would be inquiring about what he has done for enjoyment in the past. Simply offering solutions such as "get more rest" or "take breaks" may not be in alignment with this client's Recovery Lifestyle given his established Lived Identities.

However, if getting an authentic home-cooked meal from his mother is soothing, a suggestion would be for the client to pick up groceries that his mother needs to make his favorite Nigerian dish and bring his family (wife and child) along with him when he visits his parents to have a family dinner. This allows the client to see that his new Lived Identities can adapt to meet his Recovery Lifestyle while also serving as beneficial for his parents, child, and wife.

Treatment in the adult Life Stage from the CRST framework invites authentic and compassionate exploration. Life at this stage can be objectively stressful due to careers, relationships, and family transitions. It is important to validate those truths and help clients recognize that it is only a stage, and they deserve to give themselves grace as they navigate through it.

Older Adults

In a 2023 *New York Times* article, addiction medicine experts discuss the alarming rate at which the Baby Boomer generation are developing addictions. The article goes on to discuss the gap in treatment for this age group. There are currently no formal treatment approaches or interventions specifically for older adults. In this Life Stage, older adults have several established Lived Identities, but those Lived Identities are becoming less salient. The Lived Identities of parent, partner, and career at this Life Stage are often dwindling, whether it be from the passing of a partner, adult children establishing their own new Lived Identities, or retirement. Additionally, older adults have such established Lived Identities, it can be scary to think of life without them. Older adults have also lived through several generational shifts which can present as overwhelming or contribute to strong opinions about lifestyle choices. This Life Stage from the CRST framework focuses on helping clients develop new Lived Identities and increasing healthy social connections. In many cases, older adults have not recently engaged in substance use, rather, they have used substances for long periods of time, which contributes to their strong opinions about their substance use and should be considered at this Life Stage. Additionally, chronic pain plays an outsized role in addiction during this Life Stage and will be discussed in the additional considerations chapter of this book.

To work effectively with minoritized and marginalized individuals in the older adult Life Stage, understanding their established Lived Identities will assist in helping them develop new Lived Identities. For example, if an older adult speaks highly of their former career as a People Management Executive, a congruent new Lived Identity could be an AARP volunteer. If an older adult explains their disdain for having to "go out" to do things, having a bi-weekly book club or card game group may be more appropriate to develop as a part of the individual's new Lived Identity. Regardless of what the new Lived Identities are, it is important to understand what aspects of the older adult's established Lived Identities were valuable to them to assist in their discovery of new Lived Identities. My late grandfather used to tell me, "Life ain't certain, but death is for sure." What he was teaching me from that statement was something he knew to be true. His Lived Identity as a Black man born in the 1930s meant that his life was constantly in danger. Growing up in Arkansas, he experienced racism at a very young age, and had an additional Lived Identity as the son of a sharecropper. He grew up being told never to talk back to "White Folk" and to make his "own way." He taught me in this statement and through his established Lived Identities not to take life for granted, and to recognize that death is inevitable. I share this story because when working with minoritized and marginalized individuals in this Life Stage, discussing the truths of life and death are part of the process. What I mean by this is, to assist older adults in discovering new Lived Identities, you must revisit the life they have lived up to this point and help them determine how they want to live out the rest of their lives. What new Lived Identities do they want to experience? How do they want to be understood and seen in the world at this Life Stage?

Life and death can be uncomfortable topics to discuss for providers, however, for minoritized and marginalized individuals in this Life Stage, it is less uncomfortable for them than it is for you. It is likely that their minoritized and marginalized Lived Identities forced them to face the concept of death and dying far sooner and more frequently than their sessions with you. From the CRST framework, to help older adults discover new Lived Identities, you must be willing to discuss life and death as objective truths. The humanity in discussing life and death at this life stage sheds light for the individual on their Lived Identities in relation to their substance use and provides them with the hope that they have an opportunity to develop new Lived Identities. It also allows them to acknowledge their established minoritized and marginalized Lived Identities and how those identities informed their perspective on life. This information is valuable in the development of a sustainable Recovery Lifestyle for this Life Stage.

Recovery Lifestyle

Lifestyle is defined as how a person lives. It encompasses several aspects of human thought and behavior. Recovery Lifestyle is defined within the CRST framework as the way an individual thinks, feels, and perceives substance use and recovery. Stated differently, Recovery Lifestyle is how an individual lives in the context of substance use and recovery. An individual's Recovery Lifestyle informs how the individual approaches treatment and it is intended to drive their goals in recovery. In the CRST framework, Recovery Lifestyle is in place to align an individual's treatment plan with their lifestyle productively. The Recovery Lifestyle is the part of the CRST framework that gives individuals hope and encouragement in themselves and their abilities. The Recovery Lifestyle concept is influenced by Dr. Boyd-Franklin's multisystems approach. Like the multisystems approach, Recovery Lifestyle involves community support in the treatment process. Family, chosen family, spiritual or religious communities, extra-curricular groups, and social service systems all play a role in the development of an individual's Recovery Lifestyle as well as the execution of an individual's goals from the perspective of their Recovery Lifestyle. In some cases, Recovery Lifestyle may include Harm Reduction, which will be discussed in more detail in Chapter 8.

As stated in Chapter 6, Recovery Lifestyle is informed by an individual's Lived Identities. The relationship individuals have to their substance, and substance use in general, are informed by their experiences, familial perceptions, and societal influences. An individual's perception of substance use also develops from a combination of their experiences, familial perceptions, and societal influences. In the CRST Framework, an individual's Recovery Lifestyle is informed by the various people and systems with which they interact. The example of Joseph from Chapter 6 demonstrates how one's Recovery Lifestyle is developed. Some of Joseph's Lived Identities were Indigenous, caregiver, and Gen Z. Joseph's family perception of substance use was centered around plant medicines, and Joseph's generation identity of Gen Z influenced a "sober curious" mindset. Joseph's identity as a caregiver presented a level of responsibility and duty to the family that Joseph took seriously. As a result, Joseph's initial Recovery Lifestyle is such that his perception of substances was that they provide healing. This perception is influenced by his Indigenous identity and the perceptions of substances from his family. His relationship with substances was mainly positive, as he had not had any issues with substances and his mother uses substances for pain. His feelings toward substances are neutral, given his curiosity about sobriety.

Joseph's Recovery Lifestyle overall is neutral. Joseph does not need to use substances, but the sober curiosity warrants further exploration of how Joseph would like to experience substances in life. Additionally, given the perception Joseph's family has regarding substances, if Joseph shares that he wants his Recovery Lifestyle to reflect an abstinent lifestyle, exploring how that looks within his life as it pertains to his hobbies and social circles would be beneficial in assisting Joseph develop his Recovery Lifestyle. Ultimately, the goal of the provider in the context of Recovery Lifestyle in the CRST framework is to help clients discover how they think, feel, and perceive substance use. Providers are also responsible for assisting clients in identifying how they *want* to think, feel, and perceive substance use. This information will inform how you and the client develop a sustainable Recovery Lifestyle.

Relationship to Substance

In the previous example, Joseph had a neutral relationship with substances. There were no glaring feelings in either direction, with some passive thoughts of curiosity about sobriety. In many cases though, individuals have strong positive and negative relationships with substances. Some individuals have negative relationships with their substance due to the harm they have experienced or contributed to because of their substance use. Others feel like they have no control when they use substances or do not feel like "themselves." There are other individuals who have zero interest in abstaining from substances and have very positive feelings about substances. This may be due to how substances assist in numbing an emotional or physical pain. It could also be due to substances being associated with celebrations or part of normal family social gatherings. For any number of reasons, individuals have an emotional connection to substance use in part because of the connection between their substance use and their Lived Identities.

This is why the relationship to substances is an important component of the Recovery Lifestyle portion of the CRST framework. The emotional connection an individual has to the substance they are using, whether positive or negative, is strong. Consider an intimate partner relationship for example. Two individuals spend a lot of time together and develop an intimate relationship. They share emotional vulnerabilities with one another, engage in activities together, and eventually elicit strong emotions from each other due to their developed relationship. Their understanding of relationships influences how they behave in their relationship. For example, they believe spending significant amounts of time together is indicative of a good relationship, so they live and work together. They show affection in public because they perceive that behavior to be necessary to show love. They use labels like "I am [insert name's] girlfriend." They develop their "relationship lifestyle" based on their experiences of relationships and perceptions of what relationships should look like. If this couple breaks up, because of how close they became, it is extremely challenging. This former couple now experiences loneliness, sadness, isolation, and grief. Taking their behaviors as a couple and their perceptions of relationships one approach may be to encourage them to seek out platonic social gatherings. Another intervention may be to help them re-discover themselves as individuals instead of someone's partner. Eventually, they develop a lifestyle of spending time with friends, enjoying social gatherings as an individual, and learning about themselves as an individual. There is no need to challenge their enjoyment of public displays of affection (PDA), or their desire to spend lots of time with their partner. Instead, understand their lifestyle and identities to promote wellness as it is defined by them in a productive manner.

Like this relationship example, an individual who has a strong established relationship with substances and an existing substance use lifestyle would benefit from goals that reflect understanding of that lifestyle. Recovery Lifestyle in the CRST framework uses the individual's existing substance use lifestyle to inform more productive and balanced Recovery Lifestyle. If someone has a strong need to identify as an "addict," an intervention that is in alignment with their Recovery Lifestyle would be to explore other aspects of their identity that they may want to have as more of a central focus. This does not require them to no longer identify as an "addict," it simply expands their Recovery Lifestyle to develop a desire to have more identities. It is important not to underestimate the power of relationship to substances. Forcing someone to engage in a lifestyle that is not consistent with their lifestyle is where current substance use treatment fails. Recovery Lifestyle in the CRST framework opens the door for non-judgmental exploration and serves as building blocks for a sustainable and culturally responsive recovery lifestyle.

Community Support

Community support is a major component of an individual's Recovery Lifestyle because if it is in alignment, recovery maintenance is much easier than if it is not in alignment. Community support can be any individual, community, or system entity that an individual is in frequent relationship with and feels safe around. Safety within the context of community support can make or break an individual's Recovery Lifestyle because the community support is who the individuals spend the most time with. If everyone in an individual's family smokes cannabis, abstaining from cannabis effectively means stay away from your family. This is not reasonable, realistic, or culturally responsive. The CRST framework encourages adaptation as a more culturally responsive approach rather than abstinence alone. Abstinence is possible through the *adaptation* of an individual's lifestyle if abstinence is a desired part of an individual's Recovery Lifestyle. Continuing with the example of an individual whose family smokes cannabis, the individual in treatment has thoughts and feelings about cannabis that differ from their family that are influenced by what the client has observed in their family members who use cannabis. The client does not want to become "like them" but enjoys family gatherings. The client struggles with attending family gatherings due to excessive cannabis use. The client's desired Recovery Lifestyle is to be around family regardless of their cannabis use. The larger Recovery Lifestyle goal is that client wants to be unbothered by cannabis use rather than avoidant of cannabis use by others.

Understanding the makeup of the family gatherings are an important part of assisting in the development of a sustainable and culturally responsive Recovery Lifestyle. An adaptation of this client's lifestyle that is in alignment with their Recovery Lifestyle would be to start with attending family gatherings for short periods of time, and moving to different areas where the individual can be helpful, when a family member begins to smoke. The client would also identify family members, chosen family members, or other supporters to share their Recovery Lifestyle goals with, so those individuals can offer support in the moment. For example, if the individual is outside and a family member begins smoking, the individual can go inside and help prepare food, watch family children, or run to the store for last minute items. If there are no alternative activities to engage in, the individual can pull their supporter to a different area of the gathering to talk without isolating themselves. The time limit on attendance at the family gathering allows the individual to spend time with family, and gauge how long the individual can be at the family gathering "unbothered." The provider would assist the client in building on the amount of time at the family gathering by identifying activities at family gatherings that don't involve only engaging with family members who smoke cannabis. In this example, the goal of the individual's Recovery Lifestyle is to continue living their life and be unimpacted by the substance use of others. The focus is adaptation as a path to abstinence.

The example focuses on one aspect of the individual's Recovery Lifestyle as it pertains to community support, but it is important as a clinician to also help the client identify Lived Identities that promote the individual's Recovery Lifestyle. For example, if this same client enjoys playing sports but is not part of a social sport community, there may be an opportunity for the individual to further explore their Lived Identity as an athlete. Additionally, system entities such as where the client works or goes to school may offer opportunities for the client to explore other Lived Identities that promote their desired Recovery Lifestyle of being unimpacted by substance use. Something as convenient as volunteering on weekends at their local YMCA or animal shelter can foster Lived Identities of "helper." As a provider, your efforts as they relate to helping clients develop a Recovery Lifestyle that is in alignment with the client's lifestyle, will focus on learning the client's existing lifestyle, helping the client identify what they want their lifestyle to look like, and helping them adapt their existing lifestyle to become their desired lifestyle.

Substance Perceptions

How an individual perceives substances also influences their Recovery Lifestyle due to lack of information or misinformation about substances. Cannabis is illegal at the federal level, but the perception of your client is that cannabis is harmless. Fentanyl is a legal and prescribed medication, but your client's perception is that it is the drug that kills. Your client has such strong perceptions about these two substances that she is willing to smoke cannabis while pregnant but has "refuse all meds" in her birth plan because she knows fentanyl is a medication given after delivery. Her perceptions of substances influence her use and will influence her Recovery Lifestyle. This is where systems and providers can work together and efficiently to provide culturally responsive substance use treatment and build sustainable Recovery Lifestyles.

Substance perceptions often come from societal depictions of substance use and Lived Experiences. As such, it is imperative to provide psychoeducation in this portion of the CRST framework. What makes this unique though, is the way in which psychoeducation is delivered. In the CRST framework, psychoeducation needs to be delivered based on the individual's Recovery Lifestyle. "Did you know cannabis can cause popcorn lung?!" is not going to get you anywhere with an individual whose Recovery Lifestyle includes concepts like "alcohol is worse than cannabis." Instead of attempting to scare, intellectualize, and patronize individuals from minoritized backgrounds out of substance use, take time to understand why they believe their ideas about substance use. Understanding will assist you as a provider in integrating that understanding into the client's Recovery Lifestyle.

You have a client who identifies as a Black man and smokes cigarettes. You have been working tirelessly to help him understand the harmful effects of menthol cigarettes. You tell him about the disproportionate rates of lung cancer deaths in Black men. You talk about how nicotine companies are targeting Black people and he is giving his money to these companies and buying into their schemes. To no avail, your client is not interested in abstaining from smoking cigarettes. Implementing the Recovery Lifestyle portion of the CRST framework with a client like this looks like understanding his perception of cigarettes. This client tells you he has no intention of abstaining from smoking cigarettes. You ask, "what do you think about cigarettes?" He tells you that his favorite uncle smoked this specific brand when he was little, and he always wanted to be like this uncle. He shares with you; this uncle always took care of him when he was "getting into trouble" and he respected this uncle tremendously. Then you ask, "what is your relationship like with this uncle now?" Your client says flat out, "He's dead. He was in the streets, that's how he always caught me and took care of me when I was doing things I wasn't supposed to be doing. What's a cigarette going to do to me that a gun hasn't done to my people?"

Now you understand the perception your client has about cigarettes. He sees them as something people who are respected and appreciated have. You also now have knowledge that your client's concern is not about getting lung cancer, it is about getting shot. All this information funnels into the client's Recovery Lifestyle. Instead of trying to get him to stop smoking cigarettes, help him explore his identity as a Black man. Help him explore the possibility of an identity as a respected Black man in his community and what that might look like for him. Systemically, this type of information can inform robust and impactful psychoeducation for the communities served by your organization. A community outreach program might be to partner with the Big Brother/Big Sister organizations to encourage individuals in the community to become Big siblings. The Big siblings become respected adults in their community and develop intrinsic motivation to reduce their substance use in favor of being a good example. The core of the CRST framework is Lived Identity. Helping your client develop new Lived Identities within their Recovery Lifestyle and using your understanding of their substance perception will help create and sustain their Recovery Lifestyle.

Systemic Impact

The Systemic Impact portion of the CRST framework highlights various aspects of society as they relate to substance use treatment for minoritized and marginalized individuals. Social context, historical barriers, and systemic oppression make up Systemic Impact. Lived Identities, Life Stage, and Recovery Lifestyle all relate directly to the individual, but Systemic Impact looks at the role external factors have in substance use treatment for minoritized and marginalized individuals. This section of the CRST framework is intended primarily for the provider to develop an understanding of the multifaceted nature of substance use treatment. This includes provider biases, social service systems, and the criminal justice system. Systemic Impact also highlights the role systems play in contributing to the recovery of minoritized and marginalized individuals. The term "impact" is used intentionally instead of "barriers" to accurately reflect that there are productive AND unproductive facets of systems that contribute to substance use and recovery. The significance of Systemic

Impact is why the first half of the book is rooted in providing historical and cultural context. Chapters 1 through 6 outline the Systemic Impact related to substance use and recovery for minoritized and marginalized communities. This section will focus more on how to utilize Systemic Impact as part of the CRST framework.

Systemic Impact allows providers to validate the impact that systems have had on the Lived Identities of minoritized and marginalized individuals related to their substance use, substance use treatment, and recovery. Systemic Impact is also present in the CRST framework as a call to action for organizations to develop culturally responsive programs using this framework to increase access to equitable and culturally responsive substance use treatment for minoritized and marginalized individuals. The goal of Systemic Impact is to create an opportunity for providers to adopt a strengths-based approach, while simultaneously understanding the Systemic Impact present in substance use treatment for these populations.

Social Context

Helms (1990) initiated the development and facilitated the understanding of race as a social construct. This means that the concept of race and racial identities are constructed from societal interpretations of privileged groups. These societal interpretations are then used to create a social hierarchy in which minoritized individuals were at the bottom. Because racism is so ubiquitous, it is critical to acknowledge in the social context of culturally responsive substance use treatment.

Social context identifies how racism and provider bias hinder substance use treatment of minoritized and marginalized individuals. This concept in the CRST framework allows providers to take inventory of their biases and acknowledge the role racism plays in the lack of access to equitable substance use treatment. The purpose of providers taking inventory of their biases is to reduce substance use treatment stigma through addressing and challenging those biases. In the CRST framework, this should be done in multidisciplinary team meetings, clinical consult groups, and supervision. Everyone carries bias. Period. Cultural humility in this area is key to effectively recognizing and addressing biases. Checking and addressing provider bias is a critical component of Systemic Impact. Providers represent the system, whether it is the system in which they work, or their own system within their private practice, seeing a whole person and removing labels placed on them by society provides space for them to name their own Lived Identities. This helps to build a solid therapeutic foundation at the direct care level of treatment and promotes the development of a systemic norm for challenging and addressing racial as well as other forms of bias.

Another component of social context that needs to be considered by providers is the use of recovery communities as supplemental to treatment. Chapter 5 discusses the benefits and limitations of recovery communities for the purpose of this portion of the CRST framework. Recovery communities are useful and valuable for many individuals in recovery. Ensuring that you are following the CRST framework, any suggestion of involvement in recovery communities should be informed by the client's Lived Identities, Life Stage, and Recovery Lifestyle. Recovery communities can be harmful to individuals from minoritized and marginalized populations. Ensuring that providers receive input from their clients regarding recovery meetings is imperative and thinking creatively about ways individuals can build community based in the CRST framework will assist in this process.

Historical Barriers

Systemic Impact also requires providers and organizations to assess how historical barriers have contributed to an individual's lack of progress in recovery. Then, using this information, providers and organizations have a responsibility to shift and address those barriers in ways that contribute to recovery for minoritized and marginalized individuals. Labels such as "med-seeking" or "manipulating" often are attributed to behaviors of minoritized individuals in treatment, leading to premature termination in treatment or treatment "non-compliance." Additionally, existing treatment approaches focus on the "motivation" of an individual and ignore Systemic Impact, leading providers to attribute behaviors of minoritized individuals to "lack of motivation." Historical barriers in the CRST framework challenge the "lack of motivation" narrative and provide a more comprehensive understanding of an individual's progress in treatment.

For example, an individual who was incarcerated in the 1990s because of the crack epidemic (combination of history and systemic oppression), is released from prison. He has few job skills, and no concept of the way technology has advanced. His treatment while in prison was limited because his priority was not getting killed or raped. He currently has no job and does not know where to start. He frequently misses appointments due to transportation difficulties and prioritizing finding reliable sources of income. The client is not making progress in treatment in part due to his basic needs not being met. Historical barriers have contributed significantly to his inability to secure reliable work. He is not "unmotivated," his priorities are different. In this example, the provider would prioritize assisting the client in identifying his strengths and interests, which would help him discover a job he would like or skills he needs to secure a job he would like. A few ways treatment programs and organizations committed to developing culturally responsive programs would do this are by utilizing groups to focus on building job skills, enhancing their case management/recovery coach/peer advocate programs to assist individuals in completing job applications and identifying potential job opportunities, and providing work training opportunities in the profession of substance use treatment if individuals are able to maintain sobriety for a certain period of time. There are several ways for treatment programs and organizations to develop culturally responsive programs within the limitations of their system, but proper program evaluation would be essential to adapt programs within the confines of their payor requirements. Additionally, discharging patients based on their attendance alone disproportionately impacts minoritized and marginalized individuals due to historical barriers and systemic oppression. Changing discharge policies to be more culturally responsive is another component of the Systemic Impact within the CRST framework.

Systemic Oppression

This book was developed due to the seemingly insurmountable weight systemic oppression places on minoritized and marginalized individuals seeking substance use treatment. As mentioned, the emphasis of Systemic Impact in the CRST framework is for providers, programs, and organizations to recognize and act in changing the way systems address substance use treatment for minoritized and marginalized populations. Systemic oppression in the CRST framework refers to the covert and systemic ways individuals are hindered from accessing treatment. The primary example of this is insurance and insurance policies. At face value, insurance might not seem oppressive. Insurance companies are large systems that function based on the hope that individuals do not have issues. Insurance incentives for hospitals and clinics that provide care are often related to prevention metrics. If a certain percentage of individuals who carry certain insurance coverage attend "well visits," the hospital or clinic can collect a financial incentive to help fund programs. However, if those hospitals or clinics experience an influx of patients with "expensive" conditions, they are penalized by the insurance provider, or they just don't receive anything. The system is flawed, and it breeds subconscious resentment from providers because they are being punished for doing their jobs. This then leads to unjust treatment toward patients commonly referred to as "frequent flyers," but it does nothing to help people who need culturally responsive care.

It is important for providers and organizations to consider this when suggesting treatment options or follow-up care for minoritized individuals.

As discussed in Chapter 6, insurance coverage for substance use treatment is inequitable. The CRST framework as it pertains to these inequities requires systemic collaboration. Large systems providing services are responsible for connecting with community-based organizations to increase treatment access and build an ecosystem within the community. These partnerships and collaborations extend to resource-based entities such as Departments of Public Transportation to increase access to transportation and Local Libraries to promote free and reduced-fee access to technology. The CRST framework promotes developing an inclusive infrastructure between organizations to treat the whole person while simultaneously reducing the systemic barriers faced by minoritized and marginalized individuals.

Overall, the Culturally Responsive Substance Use Treatment (CRST) Framework is intended to address all aspects of the individual and the systems that impact the individual. It is for providers to take an active and culturally humble role in the way they provide treatment, and it is for organizations to shift operations to more inclusivity and equity. It is important to note that each portion of the framework may be different for the client depending on the other portions. The CRST framework is designed to be flexible enough to be used for the unique issues faced by minoritized and marginalized individuals and structured enough to be used across systems. Additionally, the CRST framework can be adapted for use with individuals who are not part of a marginalized or minoritized group, but consultation and training in adaptation would be necessary. Every section together will inform your treatment plan, your treatment approach, and your overall conceptualization of substance use from a culturally responsive lens.

References

Adames, H. Y., Chavez-Dueñas, N. Y., & Jernigan, M. M. (2023). Dr. Janet E. Helms: Envisioning and creating a more humane psychological science, theory, and practice. *American Psychologist, 78*(4), 401–412. 10.1037/amp0001037

Boyd-Franklin, N. (1989). *Black families in therapy: A multisystems approach.* Guilford Press.

Helms, J. E. (Ed.). (1990). *Black and White racial identity: Theory, research, and practice.* Greenwood Press.

Helms, J. E., & Cook, D. A. (1999). *Using race and culture in counseling and psychotherapy: Theory and process.* Allyn & Bacon.

Span, P. (2023, July 9). The hidden epidemic of substance abuse among seniors. *The New York Times.* https://www.nytimes.com/2023/07/09/health/seniors-substance-abuse.html?smid=tw-nythealth&smtyp=cur

Chapter 8

Culturally Responsive Harm Reduction

Harm reduction is a polarizing concept in part due to the lack of consistency in the conceptualization of substance use, as mentioned in previous chapters. As a result, it is critical for this book to outline harm reduction and why it is polarizing in the profession. There are multiple historical points in which harm reduction practices are utilized. Maia Szalavitz's book, *Undoing Drugs: The Untold Story of Harm Reduction and the Future of Addiction*, is a common origin story for harm reduction. In the book, Szalavitz shares that providing sterile equipment and psychoeducation regarding substance use to individuals who used substances prevented the HIV epidemic in Liverpool, England. The National Harm Reduction Coalition identifies the Black Panther Party's survival programs in the 1960s as one of the early uses of harm reduction. In the Substance Abuse and Mental Health Services Administration's (SAMHSA, 2021) release of their Harm Reduction Framework, the Key Milestones in Harm Reduction section classifies the "war on drugs" and the HIV/AIDS epidemic of the 1980s as the emerging time for harm reduction. Although these are all true instances of harm reduction, the lack of consistency in even its origins speaks to the need for systems and providers to get on the same page about harm reduction.

In 2021, SAMHSA, in partnership with the Center for Disease Control and Prevention (CDC) hosted the first federal Harm Reduction Summit. Out of this summit came a formal definition of harm reduction for agencies to follow, as well as a formal harm reduction framework. The definition of harm reduction per SAMHSA is

> *a practical and transformative approach that incorporates community-driven public health strategies—including prevention, risk reduction, and health promotion—to empower PWUD and their families with the choice to live healthy, self-directed, and purpose-filled lives. Harm reduction centers the lived and living experience of PWUD, especially those in underserved communities, in these strategies and the practices that flow from them.*

DOI: 10.4324/9781032708829-8

The framework has 6 pillars, 12 principles, and 6 core practice areas for organizations to follow.

The National Harm Reduction Coalition defines harm reduction as

a set of practical strategies and ideas aimed at reducing negative consequences associated with drug use. Harm Reduction is also a movement for social justice built on a belief in, and respect for, the rights of people who use drugs.

These two definitions speak to the challenge of getting on the same page. To start, SAMHSA definition's use of "especially those in underserved communities" is a bit patronizing when compared to the definition provided by the National Harm Reduction Coalition, which more appropriately states that harm reduction aims to "reduce negative consequences associated with drug use." The SAMHSA definition subtly perpetuates the stigma of substance use, by giving individuals a "choice" to live a healthy life. The significance of increasing access to harm reduction materials is highly beneficial from the SAMHSA definition, as it can serve as a guide for organizations and promotes institutional change in favor of harm reduction, however, the National Harm Reduction Coalition definition is more person-centered, de-stigmatizing, and still manages to address the need to dismantle systemic oppression.

It is not uncommon for government agencies to be proud of their efforts toward reducing health disparities, but actions through policy change and funding redistribution are needed more than a noble definition. Additionally, separating the behavior from the person is what differentiates the two definitions, and it is what makes the National Harm Reduction coalitions definition more de-stigmatizing for the substance use treatment world overall. When people think about harm reduction, they often think initially about providing sterile equipment to individuals using intravenous substances, providing overdose prevention medication, or providing substance test strips for individuals to check the contents of their substance. In many cases, there are also tried and true harm reduction treatment approaches that are well integrated into the medical profession. An example of this would be tobacco cessation treatment. In January 2014, the Affordable Care Act that mandated Medicaid to provide insurance coverage for smoking cessation medications went into effect. Bailey et al. (2016) conducted a study showing that this insurance coverage contributed to a 40% increase in the odds of an individual no longer smoking compared to their uninsured counterparts. This is a direct result of a harm reduction approach that is integrated into the medical profession and has penetrated institutional barriers to treatment. Unfortunately, we have known for decades that nicotine is addictive and yet, it was not until 2014 that insurance companies were required to cover treatment costs for this addiction. This example points to the disagreement at a systemic level about harm reduction treatment.

There is also unequal emphasis on what warrants harm reduction. Clearly, there are harm reduction approaches for substances that are used intravenously and substances that can lead to rapid overdose, but this is not the case for substances that can cause significant harm over time, like cannabis and alcohol. Policies and initiatives are not geared toward cannabis cessation or alcohol reduction. We don't see medical providers handing out non-alcohol beer like we see them handing out fentanyl test strips. As noted in previous chapters, there is a societal perspective about which substances truly "cause harm" and those are the substances that get the harm reduction interventions. Systems more readily adopt the harm reduction concept if it targets heroin use or methamphetamine use, but the same cannot be said for cannabis use. This discrepancy, rooted in societal perceptions, contributes to the inconsistency of harm reduction adoption across systems and industries. Expanding the reach of harm reduction to include all substances and implementing harm reduction beyond the substance are what make harm reduction culturally responsive.

Why? Harm Reduction

Daniel is an 18-year-old cis-gendered male with he/him pronouns. He grew up in a household where his parents made breakfast every day. Once Daniel graduated from high school, he was excited about living on his own. However, when he moved out of his parent's home and into his own home, he realized he had to make his own breakfast. This was challenging for Daniel because he has seen his parents cook, but he was never expected to cook for himself. As a result, Daniel started out on his own by purchasing pre-made breakfast items. After he felt more adjusted to living on his own, every Saturday, he started attempting to make his own breakfast. Initially, he burned his breakfast items and cooked inedible meals, but he practiced every Saturday. After a while, he began to make breakfast items that were edible, and eventually, breakfast items that he enjoyed and that reminded him of home. Daniel began cooking breakfast for himself daily, and even inviting his parents over for breakfast on Saturdays.

You might be wondering, "what does this have to do with harm reduction?" The concept is the same. When someone is actively engaged in substance use and substance use is a strong Lived Identity, abstinence is a sharp adjustment with no acknowledgment of the need for the development of a Recovery Lifestyle. In Daniel's case, going from receiving a ready-made breakfast every day to nothing mimics having a substance every day to no longer having that substance. In Daniel's case, the "harm reduction" approach was obtaining pre-made breakfast items, then attempting to make breakfast on his own on Saturdays, then expanding to making breakfast daily. Harm reduction can serve as a gradual shift in behavior that promotes an alternative behavior which improves a person's daily functioning. If you are a prescribing provider, you would not recommend your patient completely stop a medication they've been taking for an extended period. The same considerations should be made for individuals who have substance use conditions.

The simple answer to why harm reduction should be a standard practice in substance use treatment is that harm reduction focuses on the individual needs of someone who uses substances, in other words, meeting them where they are. (Marlatt, 1996). Additionally, the research has clearly and unequivocally demonstrated the effectiveness of harm reduction as a best practice (Des Jarlais, 2017; Hawk et al., 2017; SAMHSA, 2023). The goal of harm reduction is to "reduce the negative consequences associated with" substance use. Unfortunately, despite the research and the federal support for harm reduction as an approach to treatment, many healthcare systems and treatment organizations still require abstinence for participation in their programs. Residential treatment facilities for individuals with substance use disorders and co-occurring mental health disorders discharge individuals if they have a detected drug test. This disconnect is fundamentally rooted in the arbitrary separation of public health and mental health. The focus of substance use is different between the two professions. Public health professionals conceptualize substance use as part of a larger community issue influenced by Social Determinants of Health. As such, their approach to substance use is more in alignment with harm reduction approaches of meeting people where they are. Mental health professionals conceptualize substance use as a medical condition, yet harm reduction treatment interventions are not commonly implemented. Consider the definition of addiction as posed by the American Society of Addiction Medicine,

Addiction is a treatable, chronic medical disease involving complex interactions among brain circuits, genetics, the environment, and an individual's life experiences. People with addiction use substances or engage in behaviors that become compulsive and often continue despite harmful consequences. Prevention efforts and treatment approaches for addiction are generally as successful as those for other chronic diseases.

Although SAMHSAs still got work to do to keep from perpetuating institutionalized racism, at least there is an acknowledgement of meeting individuals where they are and utilizing community collaboration to address substance use. Minoritized and marginalized individuals are disproportionately impacted by substance use, especially intravenous substance use. As such, it is not only objectively beneficial to adopt harm reduction strategies, but also one of the most effective ways to move toward equity in substance use treatment. Public Health and mental health should not be this divergent when it comes to treatment approach. Increased collaboration between these professions through harm reduction strategy development is an aspect of the Systemic Impact portion of the CRST framework that promotes culturally responsive substance use treatment. Public Health initiatives in collaboration with mental health systems and insurance companies have a positive System Impact for minoritized and marginalized individuals in substance use treatment. This approach encompasses culturally responsive harm reduction because it addresses their Lived Identity needs by meeting them where they are, helps with the development of their Recovery Lifestyle for sustainability, and is informed by their Life Stage.

Additionally, harm reduction is beneficial for improved treatment outcomes overall. If substance use programs and residential treatment programs adopted a harm reduction approach to cannabis and alcohol like they have with smoking cessation, individuals would stay in treatment. They would be able to develop their Recovery Lifestyle while having support from their program. Imagine a client comes to a residential treatment program due to alcohol use. In the treatment program, the individual is required to attend groups, individual therapy, and complete routine drug tests. Another requirement of the program is that the individual maintains sobriety. The individual does not maintain sobriety and is kicked out of the program. The individual returns to their outpatient provider and continues to drink alcohol.

The same scenario from a harm reduction approach would be the following: The individual enters the residential treatment program, and the requirements are the same, apart from maintaining sobriety. The client meets with their therapist and discusses frequency of alcohol use and challenges with abstaining from alcohol use. The therapist offers the following harm reduction strategies: (1) the individual start with getting a glass of water before drinking and suggests the individual drink a glass of water in between alcoholic beverages; (2) the therapist provides the client with an approved 0% alcohol beverage list. The client's requirement is that if they are going to drink before group, it must be an approved 0% alcohol beverage. Each week, the client reports an increase in water consumption and 0% alcohol beverages, and a decrease in alcohol beverages. The individual is not yet abstaining from alcohol but is able to begin engaging in therapy work pertaining to underlying issues because of his decrease in alcohol consumption. Additionally, the client successfully attends groups without drinking any alcohol beverages prior. The client can identify successes in treatment and the therapist is able to identify progress in the reduction of alcohol consumption. Why harm reduction? Because it can lead to lasting recovery instead of temporary abstention.

How? Harm Reduction

As mentioned, in many cases, harm reduction is seen as the offering of sterile injection tools, increased access to overdose prevention medications, and increased access to substance test strips. However, not much happens before or after an individual receives these harm-reduction resources. There is generally an attempt made to link individuals to services, but often no consideration for how the individual will get to the appointments. For individuals who use substances that do not utilize these existing harm-reduction strategies, their only option is often an abstinence-based program. Culturally responsive harm reduction using the CRST framework takes an integrative approach that naturally incorporates harm reduction interventions within the Recovery Lifestyle section of the framework. The Systemic Impact section of the framework emphasizes how providers and agencies can leverage organizational programs to secure services and support for individuals within their communities and within systems.

An individual has been in treatment for heroin use and has "failed" to complete treatment several times because of his continued use. He has had multiple overdoses and his "pattern" is such that he ends up in the hospital, is referred back to his outpatient treatment program, and is discharged again. In his individual therapy sessions, he complains that he is not being treated fairly and no one understands what he is going through. Utilizing the CRST framework in this scenario requires first understanding his prominent Lived Identities. He shares with you that his Lived Identities are biracial, poor, and unhoused. He shares with you that he struggles with his Lived Identity of biracial because he has never felt like he "fit" anywhere. When you inquire about his desired Lived Identities, he identifies wanting to be an artist. He tells you he enjoys drawing, painting, and making music. Using the CRST framework, highlighting this desired Lived Identity as attainable for your client is critical and can be used to develop culturally responsive harm reduction strategies.

Since your client continues to use heroin, the CRST framework in the context of harm reduction implements increased use of Systemic Impact by providing the client with Narcan, substance test strips, and connecting the client with a case manager or community agency that provides sterile syringes. While the client is receiving these materials, your work would be focused on helping the client integrate their desired Lived Identity with their Recovery Lifestyle. Continuing to integrate Systemic Impact, after learning more about the client's passion for art, you suggest the client begin frequenting his local library. The local library has art activities for adults and provides a safe place for the client to go instead of where he goes on weekends to inject heroin. You can also promote the development of his desired Lived Identity and Recovery Lifestyle through exploring the idea of him taking on an apprenticeship at a tattoo shop. He can commission his artwork for tattoo art, and gain experience as an artist. You continue to explore Lived Identities with this client, allowing him the space to share the challenges of being unhoused, including understanding the circumstances around what contributed to his lack of housing, and further exploring his biracial Lived Identity. Gaining more knowledge about these Lived Identities continues to help inform the development of the client's Recovery Lifestyle.

Integration of harm reduction as a part of culturally responsive substance use treatment allows providers to understand the whole client instead of simply focusing on their substance use. Culturally responsive harm reduction requires the development of partnerships with public health agencies and a shared understanding of harm reduction. Additionally, culturally responsive harm reduction requires treatment flexibility in organizations which includes considering a reduction in substance use and a "reduction in negative consequences associated with" substance use as treatment goals.

When? Harm Reduction

Harm reduction is a valuable approach to treatment. It gives individuals more time to comprehensively work on their substance use. It also expands the conceptualization of substance use treatment to include more diverse concepts such as "sober curiosity." Harm reduction treatment emphasizes meeting individuals where they are and counts success as living a lifestyle that is in alignment with an individual's goals. So, when should harm reduction be used? The answer is always.

In the CRST framework, an individual's Recovery Lifestyle is how they want their life to look in relation to their Lived Identities and their substance use. In some cases, an individual may want to abstain from substance use and that is in alignment with their Recovery Lifestyle. In other cases, individuals may want to use certain substances and not others and that is in alignment with their Recovery Lifestyle. Then there are individuals who may want to reduce their substance use as their Recovery Lifestyle. The point is that substance use is a component of an individual's life, the emphasis on their existing Lived Identities and desired Lived Identities will inform the type of Recovery Lifestyle they have.

Harm reduction does not need to be limited to providing test strips and sterile needles. Culturally responsive harm reduction emphasizes reduction in negative outcomes of substance use while simultaneously emphasizing positive outcomes of exploring one's desired Lived Identities. Currently, harm reduction is targeted toward policy and resources, culturally responsive harm reduction expands to Lived Identities and Recovery Lifestyle. It reframes harm reduction to life enhancement for individuals who have substance use disorders. Culturally responsive harm reduction utilizing the CRST framework destigmatizes substance use and brings all aspects of the person into treatment programs, groups, and individual therapy. It holds the system accountable through providers and organizations, and it encourages collaboration across systems.

References

American Society of Addiction Medicine. (n.d.). *Definition of Addiction*. Retrieved from https://www.asam.org/quality-care/definition-of-addiction

Bailey, S. R., Hoopes, M. J., Marino, M., Heintzman, J., O'Malley, J. P., Hatch, B., Angier, H., Fortmann, S. P., & DeVoe, J. E. (2016). Effect of gaining insurance coverage on smoking cessation in community health centers: A cohort study. *Journal of General Internal Medicine*, *31*(10), 1198–1205. 10.1007/s11606-016-3781-4

Des Jarlais, D. C. (2017). Harm reduction in the USA: The research perspective and an archive to David Purchase. *Harm Reduction Journal*, *14*(51). 10.1186/s12954-017-0178-6

Harm Reduction Coalition. (n.d.). Evolution of harm reduction. Retrieved from https://harmreduction.org/movement/evolution/

Harm Reduction Principles for Healthcare Settings. (2017). *Harm Reduction Journal*, *14*(70). 10.1186/s12954-017-0196-4

Hawk, M., Coulter, R. W. S., Egan, J. E. *et al.* (2017). Harm reduction principles for healthcare settings. *Harm Reduction Journal*, *14*(70). 10.1186/s12954-017-0196-4

Marlatt, G. A. (1996). Harm reduction: Come as you are. *Addictive Behaviors*, *21*(6), 779–788. 10.1016/0306-4603(96)00042-1

Substance Abuse and Mental Health Services Administration (SAMHSA). (2021). *Harm Reduction*. Retrieved from https://www.samhsa.gov/find-help/harm-reduction

Substance Abuse and Mental Health Services Administration (SAMHSA). (2023). *Harm Reduction Framework*. Retrieved from https://www.samhsa.gov/find-help/harm-reduction/framework

Szalavitz, M. (2022). *Undoing drugs: The untold story of harm reduction and the future of addiction*. ISBN-13: 9780738285740

Psychedelic-Assisted-Treatment ... for Racial Trauma?

The coca plant, native to South America, was first used in Indigenous communities for medicinal purposes. It was further explored and the active ingredient, cocaine, was isolated by European scientists for use as a surgical anesthesia in the late 1800s (Grzybowski, 2007). Cocaine quickly became the medicine of choice for major surgeries and was heavily marketed by pharmaceutical companies to the medical industry (NIDA, 2021). Coca-Cola, which was developed in 1886 by a pharmacist, was a beverage initially containing cocaine and sugar and was only accessible from "white only" fountains and was seen as an "intellectual beverage" as noted in a 2013 *New York Times* piece. In 1899, when Coca-Cola became accessible to all, Coca-Cola went from being the "intellectual beverage" to the drink that caused "negro cocaine fiends." The same *New York Times* piece appropriately notes how Coca-Cola heavily influenced White supremacy. When White people consumed Coca-Cola, it was categorized as high social status. When Black people were given access to and consumed Coca-Cola, they were depicted as a danger to society. Dr. Carl Hart speaks to how institutionalized racism came about through cocaine drug policy in his piece written for *The Nation*. Cocaine went from being used in Indigenous communities as plant medicine, to being studied and "discovered" by European scientists, to being seen as a miracle medicine exclusively for White people, to being a substance that, if used by Black people, caused harm to Whites. At no point in time were Indigenous communities considered or consulted as the experts of medicinal use. Additionally, it was only criminalized when Black people used it.

Some might argue that cocaine is clearly identified as an illicit substance, it is not widely accepted any longer as medication (although it is still used in orthodontic surgeries), and therefore, not a sufficient example to compare to the psychedelic-assisted-treatment trajectory. Let's consider opioids as an example. Opioid medications are a class of medical and nonmedical substances, primarily prescribed for pain. These drugs

DOI: 10.4324/9781032708829-9

include, but are not limited to, oxycodone, hydrocodone, morphine, fentanyl, and heroin. In the 1990s, opioids were marketed as "non-addictive" and used to treat a wide range of pain symptoms. Oxycodone was heavily prescribed and recommended as the gold standard for pain management. The Centers for Disease Control notes that the "first wave" of the opioid crisis began with the increase of opioid prescriptions in the 1990s. What society realized rather late unfortunately, was that opioids were highly addictive, and we are now experiencing what is commonly referred to as "the fourth wave" of the opioid crisis. America is seeing an increase in illegal manufacturing of opioids and constantly evolving synthetic opioids contributing to disproportionate rates of overdose deaths in minoritized communities. This crisis is so expansive that the RAND Corporation published a 600-page book outlining "America's Opioid Ecosystem, highlighting that Opioids deserve special attention because of the multisystemic impact they have on the world of addiction as well as our national policies regarding addiction and substance use. The arc of the opioid epidemic is like the current arc we are developing with psychedelic-assisted-treatment. Psychedelics are a class of substances that can be considered medication or illicit substances. There is excitement around the prospect of psychedelics serving as "miracle drugs" for mental health and substance use disorders. If we do not begin the conversation about how to ensure psychedelics do not follow the same patterns of cocaine or opioids, we need to discuss how to progress intentionally, ethically, and with cultural consciousness in the research and utilization of psychedelics. These examples showcase the harm faced by minoritized communities because of systemic racism and lack of consideration for these communities in the research and development of new (and existing) medications. If we do not pay attention to this history, we are bound to repeat it with psychedelic-assisted-treatment.

A Time and Place for Everything

psychedelic-assisted-treatment (PAT) has gained significant traction over the past decade. The decriminalize nature movement, in which states such as California and Colorado have passed legislation to reduce or remove criminal penalties for the personal use of natural substances such as psilocybin and ayahuasca, also increased interest in psychedelic-assisted-treatment. Netflix and Hulu have released documentaries and mini-series about the evolution of psychedelics in medicine, chronicling the history of traditional psychedelic use in Native regions, to the early exploration of psychedelic treatment, the criminalization of psychedelics, and back to psychedelic-assisted-treatment reintroduction. Social interest in psychedelics includes the desire for an "awakening" or sometimes just a different experience. Research on psychedelics has become more robust, identifying specific compounds that interact with the brain that would make psychedelics truly safe alternative medication options.

Psychedelic Assisted Therapists are working to increase awareness of the research done on the effectiveness of psychedelic treatment with diagnoses including trauma, depression, and anxiety (Chi & Gold, 2020). There is also emerging research on the utilization of psychedelic-assisted-treatment for Obsessive Compulsive Disorder (OCD) (Rodrigues & Ribeiro, 2022). Psychedelics have also been seen as safer to use than traditionally prescribed medications, citing that psychedelics are natural substances with little to no addictive risk (Johansen & Krebs, 2015). More psychologists are conducting research that shows psychedelic effectiveness for a diagnosis such as PTSD is very promising (Wenk, 2023). Unfortunately, psychedelics have been criminalized and labeled as Schedule I substances, indicating that they have no therapeutic benefit, and as a result, have not been cleared for research to confirm or deny their potential utility.

There is definitely a time and place for psychedelic-assisted-treatment. The regulation that has kept psychedelics underground and out of labs needs to change. We do not know what we do not know, and research can help shed light on what true benefits and risks are associated with psychedelics. Furthermore, as we discuss culturally responsive substance use treatment, psychedelics as a substance, just like other prescription medications, will continue to need assessment regarding potential for abuse. We need to consider how to appropriately respond to psychedelic use for addiction and addiction of psychedelics. Additionally, we need to expand the consultation of these plant medicines to experts like Shamans and Medicine People from Indigenous communities who have been using these psychedelic plant medicines for centuries. If we target these concepts early in the development of psychedelic treatment and incorporate the expertise of historically overlooked traditional healers, we are less likely to make the same mistakes that landed us in an opioid epidemic.

Psychedelic-assisted-treatment should also be explored with caution when considering its use for psychiatric conditions. Psychedelic-assisted-treatment can be and should be used with intentionality, specifically as it pertains to culture. This means understanding and not mimicking Native healing practices and traditions that involved psychedelics. Indigenous communities have used plant medicine for centuries, yet the way psyche-delics have been understood has not included input from these communi-ties. When we consider culturally responsiveness in substance use treatment, understanding how the substance is intended to be used, from the perspective of those who are experts, is critical. This is what we do with other modern medicine, so just because a Shaman may not have an advanced Western degree does not discount their expertise in this area. It also means considering the potential harm using specific psychedelics may have on those Native communities. An example of potential harm caused by the psychedelic-assisted-treatment movement is the overharvesting of the peyote plant. The peyote is a cactus that contains mescaline; a chemical that has psychoactive properties and falls within the category of psychedelics. Its origins are Mexico, but it can also be found in Southern parts of Texas. Peyote has been used in Native American tribes and by Indigenous peoples as part of spiritual healing practices for generations. The plant is sacred and treated with respect and appreciation. Unfortunately, after its healing properties were "discovered" by Americans, this plant became overharvested, commercialized for tourists (Garcia-Navarro, 2007), and is currently on the endangered species list in the state of Texas. The communities who have used this plant as part of sacred practice for over 2,000 years now must fight to ensure it remains accessible. This example is one of many in which perceived medical advances outweigh the consideration of one's culture and cultural practice. Although there is benefit to psychedelic-assisted-treatment, and there is promise in medical advancements in this area, in order to keep from repeating history, there has to be a balance of understanding the cultural component and proceeding with intentionality.

The Problem of PAT and Racial Trauma

Various psychedelics have been used in indigenous populations for generations. The healing power of psychedelics has been documented throughout history and are well respected by the indigenous communities in which they are used. However, recently, there have been discussions regarding the utility of PAT for racial trauma. This is extremely problematic. To understand why this is an issue, we first need to understand what is being proposed.

The narrative around psychedelic-assisted-treatment is that it can cure most mental health conditions more effectively than traditional medication and, as a result, should be utilized. The purpose of this section of this chapter is not to argue or discount the potential benefits of psychedelic-assisted-treatment, as the research noted above confirms there is potential. Rather, it is intended to encourage professionals to better understand *why* using psychedelic-assisted-treatment for **racial trauma** is inappropriate, and harmful to minoritized communities, namely BIPOC communities. We need to place a hard stop on the notion that psychedelics should be used for racial trauma because frankly, attempting to use medications or psychedelics to treat racial trauma is backward.

Race-Based Traumatic Stress Theory (Carter, 2007) provided empirical evidence that supported conceptualizing race-related stress as a form of trauma. Research attempting to validate race-based trauma due to racial incidents utilized comparisons to other traumatic incidents to assist clinicians in recognizing the similarities in trauma responses that one might have to one or several race-related incidents (Polanco-Roman et al., 2016; Carter et al., 2020). The goal of drawing these comparisons was to raise awareness in the mental health profession of race-based trauma. Additionally, these comparisons validated the trauma that people of color experience based on institutionalized racism and systemic oppression. Researchers hoped to encourage providers to take race-based trauma seriously and treat it equitably. It was an attempt to give providers tools for how to *conceptualize* race-based trauma. Furthermore, this research was conducted to help promote the treatment of race-based trauma instead of dismissal of it as one's personal experience with no clinical association. (Bryant-Davis, 2007). Although there are many reasons why the notion of using psychedelics to treat race-based trauma is inappropriate, below I will explain the four that are most salient.

1   Using psychedelics to treat race-based trauma ignores the systems that perpetuate the trauma, to begin with.

Race-related traumatic experiences are vastly different from other traumatic experiences in part, due to the **reason** the traumatic incidents occur. Research shows that Black people are more likely to experience excessive use of force by police than White people due to prejudice and institutionalized racism (Moore et al., 2018; Motley et al., 2022). Research also identifies that exposure to racism has a direct impact on birthweight outcomes for Black women who are pregnant (Hilmert et al., 2014; Markin & Coleman, 2021). A study conducted by Yang et al. (2022) on anti-Asian racism and race-based stress highlighted news media related to the COVID-19 pandemic as contributing to race-based stress and trauma within the Asian community. Prejudice and Institutionalized Racism are what contribute to these examples of race-based trauma. Prejudice is what causes BIPOC individuals to experience high levels of fear and anxiety when they see a police officer, or when they are approached by law enforcement. Institutionalized Racism is what causes Black women to experience high levels of stress during pregnancy, and emotional dysregulation when in a hospital setting. The media pathologizing the entire Asian race to characterize a worldwide pandemic is what causes racial trauma. Unlike trauma caused by an individual, by combat, or any other uncommon situation, race-based trauma is institutionalized. It stems from the very foundation of American history and as a result, can be easy to miss. The institution is what needs to be corrected to address race-based trauma.

2 Race-based trauma is a repetitive experience.

Unlike other traumatic experiences, which are generally characterized as uncommon or infrequent, race-based trauma is a daily lived experience. Twenty years after 9/11, a Muslim woman recounted her experience as a child when 9/11 occurred. She recounted her feelings of fear after being called a "terrorist" while she walked with her sister to their mosque (Fam, 2021). This is not an isolated incident, and because of this formative experience, per her report, the fear of how she is perceived when wearing her Hijab is constant. The racial trauma experienced by BIPOC communities happens throughout one's life. To consider psychedelic-assisted-treatment to address this racial trauma invalidates the daily experience of BIPOC communities. These traumatic experiences occur through social media, television, and simply from existing. These encounters can be direct, in which the person has an experience like the person described above, or indirect, through experiences that occur to family members, friends, or people of a similar background whose stories make national headlines.

Racial trauma crosses generations. Colonization, slavery, and cultural appropriation have had continued lasting negative impacts on BIPOC communities (Gone, 2021). These parts of American history inform the way in which society functions. Segregation, immigration laws, children being separated from their families, and families being torn apart through deportation all constitute institutionalized racist practices in which BIPOC communities live. The laws, which inform the way our society functions, all contribute to repetitive traumatic race-related incidents. psychedelic-assisted-treatment would not contribute to the eradication of these institutional practices and as a result, does not address the trauma or the actual problem.

3 Using psychedelics to treat race-based trauma implies that the person who experienced the trauma has a "problem."

A 9-year-old girl in New Jersey was attempting to use a natural remedy to solve the lanternfly infestation in her community. She had been living in the neighborhood for 8 of the 9 years of her life and was well known by her neighbors. Despite this, her next-door neighbor called the police and reported, "There's a little Black woman walking, spraying stuff on the sidewalks and trees on Elizabeth and Florence. I don't know what the hell she's doing. Scares me, though." As a result of this phone call, the police went to investigate the situation. They saw the little girl, questioned her, and deemed there was no risk (Brown & Moges-Gerbi, 2022).

Unfortunately, after being stopped by the police, this 9-year-old child experienced a race-based traumatic incident while trying to contribute positively to her community. She was not the problem and did not have a problem, so why would any recommendation for her symptoms be medication, let alone psychedelics? Reactions of BIPOC individuals due to race-based traumatic incidents are responses to the trauma, and in many cases, necessary and protective.

The New Jersey incident is not uncommon, and far too many calls to the police result in the death of an innocent Black or Brown child. These stories are examples of indirect racial trauma. These instances are what cause BIPOC communities to be hypervigilant about their children playing outside and ensuring they are being watched by a trusted adult. These situations are what develop a protective fear of law enforcement for BIPOC communities. The race-based trauma is constant and real. People of color are still being murdered by police, being treated as less than human, and are disproportionately impacted by health disparities. Suggesting that symptoms of race-based trauma need to be addressed with psychedelics dismisses the truth behind why the symptoms exist. Suggesting that psychedelics are the answer for these race-based traumatic incidents absolves society of its responsibility to expose and eliminate racism. Further, it places responsibility on BIPOC communities to eliminate behavior that is protective and conducive to survival.

4 Using psychedelics to treat race-based trauma disregards the history of harmful experimentation on BIPOC communities.

The Tuskegee Syphilis Study occurred between the years of 1932 and 1972, in which almost 400 Black men diagnosed with syphilis, were studied under misleading and false information. Though there was treatment available for the disease, the Black participants were not informed and were not provided treatment. The participants were also misinformed about the purpose and length of the study and as a result, more than 100 men died from the treatable disease (Centers for Disease Control and Prevention, 2022). What was later discovered, is that a similar experiment was conducted from 1946 to 1948, in which Guatemalan soldiers were infected with syphilis and gonorrhea by U.S. physicians without consent per the instruction of the federal government. The rationale was that this study was done to help develop better methods for infection prevention (Tobin, 2022). Proponents of psychedelic-assisted-treatment for racial trauma note that BIPOC communities are excluded from research that can be beneficial for treatment and should be considered in early psychedelic studies (Fogg et al., 2021). However, given the history of manipulation and harm done to BIPOC communities through medical research, there does not appear to be any concern for ensuring the safety of BIPOC communities. Similar to point number 2, experimentation with BIPOC communities places blame for racial trauma on minoritized communities instead of addressing institutionalized racism.

Overall, when it comes to interventions for race-based trauma, psychedelic-assisted-treatment is not the answer. This notion has the potential to cause harm in BIPOC communities and poses a significant risk to the safety of minoritized individuals. Professionals working with people impacted by racial trauma may use a trauma framework to better *understand* the gravity of symptoms but conceptualizing racial trauma does not necessarily mean utilizing the same interventions you would for other forms of trauma. "Treatment" for race-based trauma needs to occur at a system level, through policy change, training, implementation of culturally responsive mental health treatment for professionals, and dismantling institutionalized racism (Wilcox, 2022).

Why Cannabis Isn't Part of the Conversation

There is a "simple" answer to this question: cannabis is not part of the conversation because it is not "technically" a psychedelic. Cannabis binds to cannabinoid receptors in the brain. Cannabinoid receptors are receptors within the central nervous system (the brain and spinal cord) which are responsible for things like maintaining homeostasis in the body, reflexes, and movement (Zou & Kumar, 2018). Psychedelics predominantly bind to serotonin receptors, which are responsible for carrying information between nerve cells. These receptors are more responsible for mood, digestion, and physiological processes that occur in the body. Cannabis and psychedelics can induce hallucinations and what some may call an "awakening" of the mind, yet they are discussed differently, labeled differently, and treated differently in the justice system. Because of these differences, cannabis is easily dismissed from the psychedelic definition, however, cannabis and psychedelics share in the effects they have on people, which is what makes this argument more convoluted, and removes the simplicity of the initial answer.

The term "psychedelic" sweeps up other substances that also do not meet the criteria to be defined as psychedelic, meaning they bind to other receptors in the brain. MDMA (also known as Molly or Ecstasy), for example, increases activity in dopamine, noradrenaline, and serotonin. MDMA was also completely developed in a lab and has no origins in nature. MDMA's design and what receptors it acts on almost make it more appropriately defined as a stimulant. In spite of this knowledge, MDMA is perceived as a psychedelic, but cannabis is not.

Not a Psychedelic ... . Just a Schedule I

The substance scheduling system was developed through the Controlled Substances Act (CSA) of 1970. The CSA, created under President Richard Nixon, was the catalyst that spurred the "war on drugs," criminalizing several substances that had been used for medicinal purposes in BIPOC communities for decades. Schedule I substances are not allowed to be prescribed by a physician, are seen as having a high potential for abuse, are indicated as unsafe for use even under medical supervision, and have no currently accepted medical use in treatment. Psilocybin, MDMA, LSD, marijuana (cannabis), and heroin are listed under the Schedule I category. Because of this categorization, these substances cannot be studied, used, or indicated for medical purposes. In short, psychedelics and cannabis have a similar story relating to how they were viewed in the public eye initially. With the scheduling system also came the criminalization of these substances. It is with the criminalization of these substances that we begin to see divergent paths.

According to the American Civil Liberties Union (ACLU), 52% of all drug arrests in 2010 were for marijuana (possession and sale) only. That means the other 48% of drug arrests were for all other illegal substances combined. In contrast, research done by Jones and Nock (2022) notes that "classic psychedelic substance" use is associated with lower odds of "crime arrests." These "crime arrests" include the use and or sale of "drugs." There are several questions to consider with this information. Why are psychedelics not considered drugs? Why are psychedelics being used as a treatment but marijuana is categorized as a drug? How is the possession of psychedelics not considered "criminal behavior," which includes substance possession and sale? This is where cannabis and psychedelics diverge. Psychedelics are treated as potential treatment solutions and interventions while cannabis is still treated as having "no currently accepted medical use in treatment" yet both cannabis and psychedelics are still Schedule I substances.

Additionally, though data shows that Black people and White people use marijuana at roughly the same rate, Black people are approximately 3.64 times more likely than White people to be arrested for possession of marijuana. The ACLU also found that more marijuana arrests were made in 2018 than for all violent crimes combined. The findings highlight the unconscious biases that the medical profession carries regarding marijuana and systemic racism that contributes to the disproportionate rates of incarceration due to marijuana in BIPOC communities. Culturally responsive substance use treatment is not just about treatment delivery, it is also about understanding these institutionalized forms of oppression and mischaracterization of substances.

Psychedelic-assisted-treatment is here and will continue to evolve as regulations for these substances continue to open doors for more research. It is critical that as we think about psychedelic-assisted-treatment, we ensure traditional healers are part of the conversations. It is important to develop policy that is clear and consistent, reducing the likelihood of minoritized communities being punished for the same behavior of White individuals. Programs need to ensure they are not mischaracterizing an individual's racial trauma as a product of something that individual did wrong, but instead raising awareness that racial trauma is a product of institutional and systemic issues. Additionally, consideration needs to be made for how we are categorizing psychedelics and consistency in how we address, research, and implement use of these substances should be consistent whether cannabis is included or not.

References

Alexander, M. (2013, January 28). The new Jim Crow. *The New York Times*. Retrieved from https://www.nytimes.com/2013/01/29/opinion/when-jim-crow-drank-coke.html

American Civil Liberties Union. (n.d.). *Marijuana arrests by the numbers*. https://www.aclu.org/gallery/marijuana-arrests-numbers

Brown, J. & Moges-Gerbi, M. (2022, November 23). *A neighbor's call to police on a little Black girl while she sprayed lanternflies exposes a deeper problem, mom says*. CNN. https://www.cnn.com/2022/11/23/us/lanternflies-black-girl-new-jersey-police-reaj

Bryant-Davis, T. (2007). Healing requires recognition: The case for race-based traumatic stress. *The Counseling Psychologist*, *35*(1), 135–143. 10.1177/0011000006295152

Canal, C. E. (2018). Serotonergic psychedelics: Experimental approaches for assessing mechanisms of action. *Handbook of Experimental Pharmacology*, *252*, 227–260. 10.1007/164_2018_107

Carter, R. T. (2007). Racism and psychological and emotional injury: Recognizing and assessing race-based traumatic stress. *The Counseling Psychologist*, *35*(1), 13–105. 10.1177/0011000006292033

Carter, R. T., Kirkinis, K., & Johnson, V. E. (2020). Relationships between trauma symptoms and race-based traumatic stress. *Traumatology*, *26*(1), 11–18. 10.1037/trm0000217

Centers for Disease Control and Prevention. (2022, December 5). *The Syphilis Study at Tuskegee Timeline*. https://www.cdc.gov/tuskegee/timeline.htm

Centers for Disease Control and Prevention. (2023, August 8). Opioid overdose: Understanding the epidemic. *CDC*. Retrieved from https://www.cdc.gov/opioids/basics/epidemic.html

Chi, T., & Gold, J. A. (2020). A review of emerging therapeutic potential of psychedelic drugs in the treatment of psychiatric illnesses. *Journal of the Neurological Sciences*, *411*, 116715. 10.1016/j.jns.2020.116715

Fam, M., Hajela, D., & Henao, L. A. (2021, September 6). *Two decades after 9/11, Muslim Americans still fighting bias*. Associated Press. https://apnews.com/article/September-11-Muslim-Americans-93f97dd9219c25371428f4268a2b33b4

Fogg, C., Michaels, T. I., de la Salle, S., Jahn, Z. W., & Williams, M. T. (2021). Ethnoracial health disparities and the ethnopsychopharmacology of psychedelic-assisted psychotherapies. *Experimental and Clinical Psychopharmacology*, *29*(5), 539–554. 10.1037/pha0000490

Garcia-Navarro, L. (2007, September 3). *Mexico's Peyote Endangered by 'Drug Tourists'*. National Public Radio. https://www.npr.org/2007/09/03/14064806/mexicos-peyote-endangered-by-drug-tourists

Gone, J. P. (2021). The (post)colonial predicament in community mental health services for American Indians: Explorations in alter-Native psy-ence. *American Psychologist*, *76*(9), 1514–1525. 10.1037/amp0000906

Grzybowski, A. (2007). Historia kokainy w medycynie i jej znaczenie dla odkrycia róznych form znieczulenia [The history of cocaine in medicine and its importance to the discovery of the different forms of anaesthesia]. *Klinika oczna*, *109*(1–3), 101–105.

Hallifax, J. (2022, Sept. 2). *Is marijuana a psychedelic?* Psychedelic Spotlight. https://psychedelicspotlight.com/is-marijuana-a-psychedelic/

Hart, C. L. (2017). People are not dying because of opioids. *Scientific American*, *317*(5), 12. 10.1038/scientificamerican1117-11

Hilmert, C. J., Dominguez, T. P., Schetter, C. D., Srinivas, S. K., Glynn, L. M., Hobel, C. J., & Sandman, C. A. (2014). Lifetime racism and blood pressure changes during pregnancy: Implications for fetal growth. *Health Psychology*, *33*(1), 43–51. 10.1037/a0031160

Johansen, Ø., & Krebs, T. S. (2015). Psychedelics not linked to mental health problems or suicidal behavior: A population study. *Journal of Psychopharmacology*. 10.1177/0269881114568039

Jones, G. M., & Nock, M. K. (2022). Psilocybin use is associated with lowered odds of crime arrests in US adults: A replication and extension. *Journal of Psychopharmacology (Oxford, England)*, *36*(1), 66–73. 10.1177/02698811211058933

Mackie, K. (2008). Signaling via CNS cannabinoid receptors. *Molecular and Cellular Endocrinology*, *286*(1–2 Suppl 1), S60–S65. 10.1016/j.mce.2008.01.022

Mangini, M. (2021). A short, strange trip: LSD politics, publicity, and mythology—From discovery to criminalization. In C. S. Grob & J. Grigsby (Eds.), *Handbook of medical hallucinogens* (pp. 68–94). The Guilford Press.

Markin, R. D., & Coleman, M. N. (2021). Intersections of gendered racial trauma and childbirth trauma: Clinical interventions for Black women. *Psychotherapy*. Advance online publication. 10.1037/pst0000403

Moore, S. A., Robinson, M. M., Clayton, D., Adedoyin, A. C. A., Boamah, D., Kyere, E., & Harmon, D. (2018). A critical race perspective of police shooting of unharmed Black males in the United States: Implications for social work. *Urban Social Work*, *2*, 33–47. 10.1891/2474-8684.2.1.33

Motley, R. O., Jr., Joe, S., McQueen, A., Clifton, M., & Carlton-Brown, D. (2022). Development, construct validity, and measurement invariance of the Modified

Classes of Racism Frequency of Racial Experiences Measure (M-CRFRE) to capture direct and indirect exposure to perceived racism-based police use of force for Black emerging adults. *Cultural Diversity and Ethnic Minority Psychology.* Advance online publication. 10.1037/cdp0000525

Musto, D. F. (1999, April 14). The American Disease: Origins of Narcotic Control. *The Nation.* Retrieved from https://www.thenation.com/article/archive/how-myth-negro-cocaine-fiend-helped-shape-american-drug-policy/

National Institute on Drug Abuse. (2021, April 8). Cocaine. *NIDA.* Retrieved from https://www.drugabuse.gov/drug-topics/cocaine

Ortiz, N. R., & Preuss, C. V. (2022). Controlled substance act. In *StatPearls.* StatPearls Publishing.

Polanco-Roman, L., Danies, A., & Anglin, D. M. (2016). Racial discrimination as race-based trauma, coping strategies, and dissociative symptoms among emerging adults. *Psychological Trauma: Theory, Research, Practice and Policy, 8*(5), 609–617. 10.1037/tra0000125

Redman, M. (2011). Cocaine: What is the crack? A brief history of the use of cocaine as an anesthetic. *Anesthesiology and Pain Medicine, 1*(2), 95–97. 10.5812/kowsar.22287523.1890

Rodrigues, J., Nombora, O., & Ribeiro, L. (2022). Therapeutic potential of serotoninergic psychedelic substances in the treatment of obsessive compulsive disorder. *European Psychiatry, 65*(S1), S647–S647. 10.1192/j.eurpsy.2022.1659

Stein, B. D., Kilmer, B., Taylor, J., & Vaiana, M. E. (Eds.). (2023). *America's opioid ecosystem: How leveraging system interactions can help curb addiction, overdose, and other harms.* Santa Monica, CA: RAND Corporation. Retrieved from https://www.rand.org/pubs/research_reports/RRA604-1.html

Tobin, M. J. (2022). Fiftieth anniversary of uncovering the Tuskegee Syphilis Study: The story and timeless lessons. *American Journal of Respiratory and Critical Care Medicine, 205*(10), 1145–1158. 10.1164/rccm.202201-0136SO

Wenk, G., Chadderton, P., Golden, C., & Marano, H. E. (2023, January). *Why psychedelics are therapy's next frontier.* Psychology Today. https://www.psychologytoday.com/us/articles/202301/why-psychedelics-are-therapys-next-frontier

Wilcox, M. M. (2022). Oppression is not "culture": The need to center systemic and structural determinants to address anti-Black racism and racial trauma in psychotherapy. *Psychotherapy.* Advance online publication. 10.1037/pst0000446

Yang, J. P., Nhan, E. R., & Tung, E. L. (2022). COVID-19 anti-Asian racism and race-based stress: A phenomenological qualitative media analysis. *Psychological Trauma: Theory, Research, Practice, and Policy, 14*(8), 1374–1382. 10.1037/tra0001131

Zou, S., & Kumar, U. (2018). Cannabinoid receptors and the endocannabinoid system: Signaling and function in the central nervous system. *International Journal of Molecular Sciences, 19*(3), 833. 10.3390/ijms19030833

Chapter 10

Additional Considerations

We Don't Know What We Don't Know

What generally happens when you ask a teenager why they did something? How about when you ask them how they are feeling? Overwhelmingly, and throughout the generations, the answer is almost always "I don't know." It can come in the form of a shoulder shrug, a turned-down mouth, an "IDK" through a text, or just an audible "I don't know." Sometimes it is evident that they *do* know, and are using the common response to buy themselves time to think of a good lie. Other times, though, they really *don't* know why they did something, or how they are feeling in that moment. This phrase, commonly loathed by parents all over the world, is said in part due to the lack of frontal lobe development in an adolescent. They really do not know why they engaged in a behavior, or they really don't know how they are feeling in the moment because their brain has not developed enough for them to be able to connect their thoughts and feelings with their actions.

The same goes for culturally responsive substance use treatment. Because culture is constantly evolving, and because substances can come from nature or be developed in a lab, we really don't know what we don't know. Keeping this in mind when engaging in culturally responsive substance use treatment is critical, as it allows you to keep an open mind and continue to seek new information to help improve how you approach substance use issues. When the term "addict" became popular, we didn't know that using the term would become a heated topic of debate among professionals. We didn't know that person first language would be something that now directs the way we speak about mental health and substance use. Not knowing is normal, problems arise when a profession is not *willing* to learn. Whatever role you carry in your organization, ensure that you are seen as someone who is willing to learn. In embracing a willingness to learn, it is also important to develop a willingness to acknowledge your mistakes. When a staff member points

DOI: 10.4324/9781032708829-10

out a microaggression, or when a client reports feeling invalidated after a session, use that information to facilitate change and improve company practices as a way of acknowledging mistakes. Having this posture will be advantageous for you as you consider ways in which you can contribute to promoting an equitable and culturally responsive environment. It is also important to *hear* what is being said. An African proverb states, "Examine what is said, not who is speaking." Unfortunately, our society places value on who says what. If a well-known celebrity endorses a shoe and says it is comfortable, people are more inclined to believe the shoe is comfortable. However, if a person who is not well-known says that the same shoe is comfortable without the endorsement of the celebrity, people are less likely to believe that person. To be frank, minoritized individuals have been saying that medical and mental health treatment are inequitable for generations. Society has ignored the voices of minoritized individuals and is now being faced with the consequences of ignoring those voices. Racism exists. It doesn't exist because a White person says it exists and it doesn't exist because a Black person says it exists. It exists because that is how our country was built and that is what has been reinforced through society. Minoritized scholars have said this for decades. It is time to listen to what is being said so we can make sustainable and systemic change. The core of culturally responsive substance use treatment is *responding* to the culturally diverse needs of the clients served based on what the client identifies as their need. Believe what individuals from Minoritized and Marginalized backgrounds say when they share their difficult past experiences in treatment. Validate individuals' experiences of racism, sexism, homophobia, and whatever other -ism they share with you. Don't make the same mistakes that contributed to their lack of trust in the system or their premature termination of treatment.

We also don't know what we don't know as it pertains to the future of psychedelics. The opioid epidemic is a cautionary tale for how we should approach psychedelics differently. There is a template for what not to do and it is my hope that as we embark on this assisted treatment approach we proceed with intentionality and caution. I encourage re-reading Chapter 9 now that you have read through the framework and see how the framework informs your understanding of the chapter and its significance.

The layout of this book was very intentional, initially emphasizing historical context and highlighting aspects of substance use and life that are not commonly discussed together. This was followed by an introduction to the Culturally Responsive Substance Use Treatment (CRST) framework. There are several topics that were not addressed explicitly in this book. Substance use and substance use treatment are expansive topics and everything cannot adequately be covered well in one book. Common topics that are generally examined when discussing substance use are trauma, people with lived experience, people with chronic pain, and family members impacted by a loved one's substance use. Each of these topics can stand alone with their own book, and it is my hope that the release of this book will promote a request for more books like this to adequately address these topics, as well as topics I have not mentioned that would benefit from more integration of cultural responsiveness and substance use treatment. Additionally, the resources section of this book will also offer tools to utilize for individuals interested in learning about those well-established topics. However, there is still a need for more content to be disseminated regarding the relationship between culturally responsive substance use treatment and these topics. Culturally responsive substance use treatment is more than identifying considerations for Minoritized and Marginalized communities, it requires a comprehensive framework and that was the purpose of this book.

Culturally Responsive Advocacy

Advocacy is defined as public support for or recommendation of a particular cause or policy. A recent and applicable example of advocacy by this definition is the "Blackout Tuesday" movement. On June 2, 2020, many individuals took to their social media accounts to post a Black square. The purpose of the Black square was to represent an explicit opposition to racism. What many individuals did not know, was this initiative was started by two Black women who were music executives and the initial hashtag for the movement was #TheShowMustBePaused. The purpose of the initiative was to halt the release of music and content as a representation of the significant economic impact Black musicians and Black consumers have on the music industry. The pause of content and content purchasing was intended to represent the significance of Black lives in the country. Unfortunately, this effort quickly became misguided and damaging to the Black Lives Matter movement due to the performative efforts of White individuals (Wellman, 2022). In an attempt to be seen as an ally, but not taking the time to understand the purpose of the action, White individuals began posting Black squares and hashtagging #BlackLivesMatter. In this example, social media influencers and individuals wanting to be seen as allies posting Black squares to show public support for the Black Lives Matter movement is technically advocacy. However, instead of creating change, this action only hurt the Black Lives Matter movement and diminished its initial intent.

Culturally responsive advocacy is advocacy that **actively contributes** to social change. It requires individuals who want to advocate for social change to understand what they are supporting by doing the research. It also requires influencer allies to go beyond their social media bubble and use their platform to encourage their followers to vote for policy that will help dismantle institutional racism. It looks like individuals speaking against policy that perpetuates marginalization in their companies. Specific to substance use and substance use treatment, culturally responsive advocacy looks like being intentional about using person-first language, speaking against policy that reinforces the "Not In My Backyard" culture, and promoting harm reduction in systems. Collective action is what drives change, but a collective is made up of individuals. Your power and privilege as an individual are critical to building a more equitable society collectively.

Community Awareness and Outreach

It is easy to ignore something if it doesn't directly pertain to your life or lifestyle. It is also easy to avoid looking beyond the surface of social issues that do not directly impact your life or lifestyle. To move toward a more equitable culture and society, we must stop operating within what makes us feel comfortable. In my trainings, when I discuss cultural responsiveness, responses I get from the audience are that this concept is "too big." People become overwhelmed and the sentiment stops them from doing anything differently. Once my trainings are complete, these same individuals identify the practicality and approachability of the concepts. Sometimes community awareness looks as small as having an ally sign in your front yard. By having that sign, you are not only letting minoritized individuals know that you are safe, but you are raising awareness in your community. You are metaphorically opening the door for conversations to be had about why you have the sign and what it means. Having those conversations may be uncomfortable, but they are necessary for progress to be made. Progress in dismantling racism equals progress in everything else.

Outreach is also an important aspect of moving equity forward. Outreach may look like providing talks to your local schools, churches, or libraries about ways to support individuals with substance use disorders. Outreach is an underdeveloped approach in the mental health profession, but it is well-established in the public health sectors. Collaborating with public health organizations and promoting events hosted by public health agencies are dynamic and practical ways to contribute to outreach efforts.

Although we have a long way to go as a society toward equity, there are steps we are taking and can continue to take to keep moving forward. It is my hope that this book raises your awareness, provides you with tools and resources, and motivates you to work toward providing culturally responsive substance use treatment and mental health treatment in whatever seat you sit. I also want to remind you that treatment approaches and conceptualization are ongoing processes. As such, culturally responsive substance use treatment is ever-evolving because culture itself is ever evolving.

Reference

Wellman, M. L. (2022). Black squares for Black lives? Performative allyship as credibility maintenance for social media influencers on Instagram. *Social Media + Society*, *8*(1). 10.1177/20563051221080473

Resources

This resource list will include books that provide context regarding the significance of increasing antiracist practices and practical strategies to utilize as you work toward dismantling racism. It will also include books on trauma, lived experience, chronic pain, and families impacted by substance use.

Antiracism

- *Stamped from the Beginning: The Definitive History of Racist Ideas in America* by Ibram X. Kendi
- *How to Be a (Young) Antiracist* by Ibram X. Kendi
- *The (Young) Antiracist's Workbook* by Ibram X. Kendi
- *The Antiracism Handbook: Practical Tools to Shift Your Mindset and Uproot Racism in Your Life and Community* by Dr. Thema Bryant and Dr. Edith G. Arrington

Trauma

- *Thriving in the Wake of Trauma: A Multicultural Guide* by Dr. Thema Bryant
- *Cultural Safety in Trauma-Informed Practice from a First Nations Perspective: Billabongs of Knowledge* by Nicole Tujague and Kelleigh Ryan
- *Racial Trauma Clinical Strategies and Techniques for Healing Invisible Wounds* by Kenneth Hardy, Ph.D.

Lived-Experience

- *Punch Me Up to the Gods: A Memoir* by Brian Broome
- *Angel on My Shoulder: An Autobiography* by Natalie Cole
- *Unashamed* by Lecrae

- *God and Starbucks: An NBA Superstar's Journey Through Addiction and Recovery* by Vin Baker

Chronic Pain

- *Managing Chronic Pain in an Age of Addiction* by Akhtar Purvez, MD, and John Rowlingson, MD
- *Chronic Pain and Addiction* by M. R. Clark and G. J. Treisman

Impacted Family Members

- *Addiction Support: How to Help Your Loved One with Addiction* by Angel Ayala

Index